Discovering and Nutrition

Seventh Edition

Student Workbook

Connie R. Sasse, CFCS

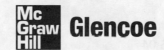

Glencoe

New York, New York   Columbus, Ohio   Chicago, Illinois   Peoria, Illinois   Woodland Hills, California

Illustrations:

Angela Burns
M.R. Greenberg
Daniel Grossman
Kelly Hinkle
Elizabeth Purcell

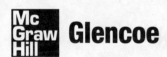

Glencoe

The **McGraw·Hill** Companies

Send all inquiries to:
Glencoe/McGraw-Hill
3008 W. Willow Knolls Drive
Peoria, Illinois 61614-1083

ISBN 0-07-861683-2 (Student Workbook)

Printed in the United States of America

1 2 3 4 5 6 7 8 9 10 009 09 08 07 06 05 04

CONTENTS

UNIT FIVE: MEALTIME

UNIT SIX: LEARNING ABOUT FOODS

UNIT SEVEN: CREATIVE COMBINATIONS

UNIT EIGHT: BAKING

CHAPTER 1

The Adventure of Food

Study Guide

Directions: Answer the following questions on the lines provided.

1. How can learning about food and nutrition help keep you healthy and active throughout your life?

_____

_____

2. Why is it important to eat a variety of nutritious foods each day?

_____

_____

3. Why is it an advantage to know how to prepare many different foods?

_____

_____

_____

4. What are four ways you will be able to use food preparation skills?

_____

_____

_____

5. What are five skills you will practice in foods class that you can use in your daily life?

_____

_____

_____

6. What are two advantages of setting goals?

_____

_____

Continued on next page

7. Compare and contrast long- and short-term goals.

_____

_____

_____

8. Describe three short-term goals that will help you accomplish the long-term goal of fixing a meal for your friends.

_____

_____

_____

_____

9. What is self-confidence?

_____

_____

10. How can studying food and nutrition help you gain self-confidence?

_____

_____

11. What is involved in becoming skillful in food preparation?

_____

_____

12. How can you measure your progress as you practice preparing food?

_____

_____

_____

CHAPTER 1

The Adventure of Food

Going for the Goal

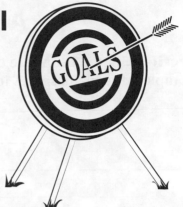

Directions: Read the goals listed below. Write "short" in the blank to the left of the goal if it is a short-term goal. Wrie "long" in the blank to the left of the goal if it is a long-term one.

_____ 1. Casey wants to finish the pillow she's sewing by this Friday.

_____ 2. Nick hopes to get at least a B on his foods test this class period.

_____ 3. Gwen is saving her money for a compact disc player.

_____ 4. Juanita wants to become an engineer.

_____ 5. Emily plans to buy new shoes after school.

_____ 6. Brandon wants to learn to make pizza from scratch in his foods class.

_____ 7. Paul plans to visit his grandmother this weekend.

_____ 8. Makayla wants to attend the local community college when she graduates from high school.

_____ 9. Joe is going to buy groceries after school.

_____ 10. Andrea has to pick up her softball uniform from her manager before the first game next week.

_____ 11. Mike wants to raise his free-throw percentage to 75 percent before the end of the basketball season.

_____ 12. Ashley wants to work as a supermarket bagger next summer.

_____ 13. Bo hopes to earn an A in his foods class this semester.

_____ 14. Lori plans to attend the football game this Friday night.

_____ 15. Kym Lee is saving money for a car of his own.

CHAPTER **1**

The Adventue of Food

A Puzzling Adventure

Directions: Listed below are clues that have to do with the adventure of food. Use each clue to complete the blank spaces in the corresponding numbered item.

1. __ **A** __ __ __ __
2. __ __ __ __ __ **D** __ __ __ __
3. __ __ __ __ __ **V** __
4. __ **E** __
5. __ __ **N** __ - __ __ __ __
6. __ __ __ __ **T** __ __ __ __
7. __ **U** __ __ __ __ __ __ __
8. __ __ __ **R** __ - __ __ __ __
9. __ __ __ **E** __

Clues

1. The study of foods could lead to this in the food industry.

2. Having this in yourself means you believe you will succeed.

3. Nutritious foods will help keep you in this condition.

4. You will work as a part of this in the foods laboratory.

5. A goal to accomplish far in the future.

6. What it will take to master food preparation skills.

7. Learning about this in foods class will help you look and feel your best.

8. A goal to be accomplished in the near future.

9. This is what a goal is like.

CHAPTER 2

Managing Your Resources

Study Guide

Directions: Answer the following questions on the lines provided.

1. What is a resource? What are the four kinds of resources?

_____

_____

_____

2. What is the relationship between resources and management?

_____

_____

3. What are personal resources? Material resources?

_____

_____

_____

4. What kinds of help can social resources provide for you?

_____

_____

5. What are five examples of resources in your community?

_____

_____

_____

6. Identify four examples of natural resources.

_____

_____

_____

Continued on next page

7. What are some ways you can use resources wisely? Which is the easiest resource to increase? Why?

_____

_____

8. Why is conserving resources important?

_____

_____

9. Give an example of how one resource can be substituted for another.

_____

_____

_____

10. List the steps in making decisions.

_____

_____

_____

11. What factors should you consider when comparing options in making decisions?

_____

_____

_____

12. What does it mean to evaluate?

_____

_____

CHAPTER 2
Managing Your Resources

Resource Match Ups

Directions: Match each resource in the left column with the correct type of resource from the right column. Write the letter of the type of resource in the space provided. Each type of resource will be used at least once.

Resource

____ 1. A free afternoon to do what you'd like

____ 2. Fuel to heat the house in winter

____ 3. A $20 bill for your birthday that you can spend any way you want

____ 4. A softball and bat

____ 5. A best friend

____ 6. The ability to change the oil in a car

____ 7. A park across the street from your home

____ 8. The energy to run three miles

____ 9. The local library

____ 10. A dishwasher

____ 11. Fresh water in the tap

____ 12. A home to live in

____ 13. Emotional support from parents

____ 14. Gasoline to run the car

____ 15. Skills to make curtains

Type of Resource

A. Material resource

B. Natural resource

C. Personal resource

D. Social resource

CHAPTER **2**

Managing Your Resources

Holly's Choice

Holly has decided to treat her friend Anna to dinner on Anna's birthday. Anna really likes Mexican food and enjoys going to the Mexican Fiesta Restaurant. Holly would like to take her there, but she doesn't have enough money. She would have to borrow some money to pay for the dinner. Holly knows how to make tacos, nachos, and enchiladas. She thinks she has enough money to buy the ingredients to cook a birthday dinner for Anna. However, she's afraid making dinner for Anna at home won't seem very festive. Use the steps in the decision-making process to help Holly make her choice. Write your answers to the questions below on the lines provided.

1. What exactly is the decision Holly is trying to make?

   _____

   _____

2. What are Holly's resources?

   _____

   _____

3. What options does Holly have?

   _____

   _____

4. What are the good and bad points of each option?

   _____

   _____

   _____

   _____

5. Which option do you think Holly should choose? Why?

   _____

   _____

6. How will Holly know whether she made the right choice?

   _____

   _____

CHAPTER 3   What About Careers?

Study Guide

Directions: Answer the following questions on the lines provided.

1. What is a career? _____

_____

_____

2. What personal qualities are the basis for a successful career?

_____

_____

3. What are three characteristics of a responsible worker?

_____

_____

_____

4. Why is the "willingness to learn" a skill you will need your whole life?

_____

_____

_____

5. Give an example of how you might use communication skills on the job.

_____

_____

_____

6. Why would a person interested in the food industry need to have computer skills?

_____

_____

Continued on next page

7. Why is teamwork an important workplace skill?

_____

_____

8. What are three ways a person can develop the qualities needed to be a successful worker?

_____

_____

9. What is an entry-level job?

_____

_____

10. What does a dietitian do on the job?

_____

_____

11. What is the overall purpose of careers in food production, processing, distribution, and marketing?

_____

_____

12. What do food service workers do?

_____

_____

CHAPTER 3

What About Careers?

Job Skills

Directions: The list below on the left describes various on-the-job activities of some of the people who work in a supermarket. Decide what ability listed in the right column is shown by the employees and write its letter in the blank to the left of the activity described.

Activities on the Job

Abilities Shown by Employees

_____ 1. Josie and Kelly worked together to refill a frozen food case.

A. Willingness to learn

_____ 2. Jeff has been asked to learn the new computer program the store is purchasing.

B. Communication skills

_____ 3. David monitors the fax and copy machines so they don't run out of paper.

C. Basic math skills

_____ 4. Meg added the receipts from six cash drawers at the end of the shift.

D. Teamwork

_____ 5. Drew wrote a report explaining the advantages of installing an automatic sprinkling system in the produce department.

E. Responsibility

F. Computer skills

_____ 6. Becka figured out a new system that made it easier to do the daily bank deposit.

G. Thinking skills

_____ 7. Marcus talked to Kelly about how important it was that she start coming in on time for her shift.

H. Management skills

_____ 8. Trey sends a report of each day's sales to the store's owner using e-mail.

_____ 9. Meg was assigned to work with the Downtown Merchants Association to plan a holiday promotion for Halloween.

_____ 10. Jeff enters each week's sale prices into the computer so the scanners will scan the correct price.

_____ 11. Becka adds up the employees' hours each week so their paychecks can be written.

CHAPTER **3**

What About Careers?

Looking at Careers

Directions: Read each situation described below. Answer the questions on the lines provided.

1. Chamique enjoys helping people. She is also very organized and likes to do things the "right" way. Her counselor suggested she consider a career as a dietitian. Chamique doesn't know much about what a dietitian does. She wonders whether it would be a good career choice for her. Do you think it might be? Why or why not?

   _____

   _____

   _____

   _____

2. Andrew wants to be a scientist. One of his hobbies is cooking. He wonders if there is any way he could combine these interests. Suggest a possible career in the food industry for Andrew and explain why it could be appropriate for him.

   _____

   _____

   _____

   _____

3. Taylor works part-time job in a restaurant while she is in school. She enjoys it a lot and thinks she might like a career in food service. She does not want to be a chef and hopes to advance beyond the customer service staff. What other career in food service might Taylor consider? What types of work would she do in that career?

   _____

   _____

   _____

   _____

Name _____ Date _____ Class Period _____

CHAPTER 4

Wellness—Your Goal for Life

Study Guide

Directions: Answer the following questions on the lines provided.

1. What is wellness?

   _____

   _____

2. What are three benefits of choosing nutritious foods?

   _____

   _____

3. Why is it not a good idea to try to achieve an "ideal" body shape?

   _____

   _____

   _____

4. What are four benefits of regular physical activity? How much physical activity provides the most benefit each day?

   _____

   _____

   _____

   _____

5. What are two ways to build strength?

   _____

   _____

6. Why is flexibility important? How can it be developed?

   _____

   _____

Continued on next page

7. What are two benefits of endurance activities?

_____

_____

_____

8. Why is sleep important to good health? How does a person know if he or she is getting enough sleep?

_____

_____

_____

9. What is a positive advantage of stress?

_____

_____

10. Give four suggestions for reacting positively to stress.

_____

_____

_____

11. What are the advantages of following a personal wellness plan now?

_____

_____

12. What kind of help can a health professional give in developing a wellness plan?

_____

_____

CHAPTER 4
Welness—Your Goal for Life

Will's Wellness Plan

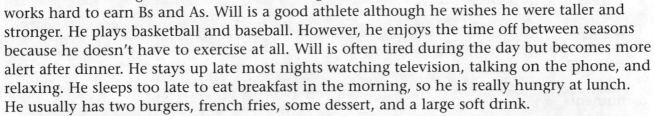

Directions: Read the case example below. On the lines provided, list six ways to increase health and wellness. Explain how well Will does on each and give a suggestion for Will to improve that part of his life.

   Will wants to major in pharmacology (far-MUH-kahl-uh-jee) when he goes to college. His parents put a lot of emphasis on getting good grades so he can attend college. Will worries about his grades and works hard to earn Bs and As. Will is a good athlete although he wishes he were taller and stronger. He plays basketball and baseball. However, he enjoys the time off between seasons because he doesn't have to exercise at all. Will is often tired during the day but becomes more alert after dinner. He stays up late most nights watching television, talking on the phone, and relaxing. He sleeps too late to eat breakfast in the morning, so he is really hungry at lunch. He usually has two burgers, french fries, some dessert, and a large soft drink.

   Will's group of friends have a lot of fun together. However, lately, a couple of guys have been drinking beer some weekends. So far, Will hasn't had any, but he knows the time is coming when he may feel pressured by his friends to drink. He wonders if he will be able to say no.

   A school dance is coming soon and Will would like to ask Courtney, a girl in his math class. He doesn't know her very well and is afraid she'll say no. Every day he works to get his courage up to ask her, but finds himself tongue-tied and ends up not asking.

1. _____

   _____

2. _____

   _____

3. _____

   _____

4. _____

   _____

5. _____

   _____

6. _____

   _____

CHAPTER **4**

Wellness—Your Goal for Life

Wellness Magic

Directions: Find the term which best fits each description. Write the number of the correct term in the space in each lettered square. If all your answers are correct, the total of the number, or the "Magic Number," will be the same in each row across and down. Write the Magic Number in the space provided.

Terms

1. stretching activity

2. aerobic activity

3. wellness

4. exercise

5. nutrients

6. sleep

7. alcohol

8. endurance

9. stress

10. muscle-building activity

A	B	C
D	E	F
G	H	I

The Magic Number is _____.

Descriptions

A. Ability to continue physical activity for a long time.
B. Good physical, emotional, and mental health.
C. Activity to firm and tone muscles.
D. Time to rid the body of waste products in the muscles.
E. Can affect reactions and judgements.
F. Helps body take in and use more oxygen.
G. Helps body be more flexible.
H. Chemicals in food that help the body work properly.
I. Emotional and physical tension.

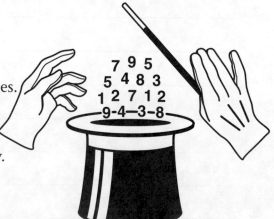

CHAPTER 5 Meet the Nutrients

Study Guide

Directions: Answer the following questions on the lines provided.

1. What are nutrients? What happens if one nutrient is missing from a person's diet?

   _____

   _____

   _____

2. Identify the six basic types of nutrients. What are the main uses of nutrients in the body?

   _____

   _____

   _____

3. What are the similarities and differences between complex and simple carbohydrates?

   _____

   _____

   _____

   _____

4. Why is fiber an important part of a healthy diet?

   _____

   _____

5. Name four jobs that fat performs in the body.

   _____

   _____

   _____

6. What are trans fats?

   _____

   _____

   _____

Continued on next page

7. How do trans fats affect the blood?

_____

_____

8. What is the role of protein in the body?

_____

_____

9. How are complete and incomplete proteins similar? How are they different?

_____

_____

_____

_____

10. Why does the body need water each day?

_____

_____

11. What is the major difference between fat-soluble and water-soluble vitamins?

_____

_____

_____

12. What role do minerals play in the body?

_____

_____

13. What are three factors that help determine how much of each nutrient you need each day?

_____

_____

14. What are phytochemicals? Why are they important?

_____

_____

Nutrient Match Up

Directions: Match each nutrient function in the left column with the correct nutrient from the right column. Write the letter of the nutrient in the space provided. Each nutrient will be used at least once.

Nutrient Functions

____ 1. Cushions vital organs

____ 2. Provides energy for the body

____ 3. Builds new cells

____ 4. Heals wounds

____ 5. Repairs injured cells

____ 6. Keeps a normal heart beat

____ 7. Keeps skin healthy

____ 8. Keeps nerves and muscles healthy

____ 9. Helps fight off disease

____ 10. Insulates body from heat and cold

____ 11. Promotes good night vision

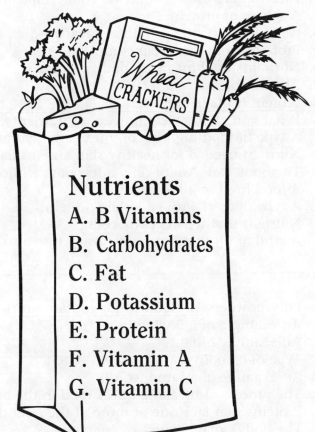

Nutrients
A. B Vitamins
B. Carbohydrates
C. Fat
D. Potassium
E. Protein
F. Vitamin A
G. Vitamin C

Discovering Food and Nutrition Student Workbook

CHAPTER 5

Text Pages 34-45

Meet the Nutrients

Puzzling Over Nutrients

Directions: Fill in the crossword puzzle by placing the answer to each clue in the appropriate space.

Across

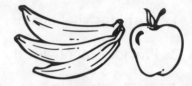

1. Fats that are usually solid at room temperature.
7. A source of protein.
8. A food that contains natural sugars.
9. Proteins from this are incomplete.
10. Nutrients used for many body processes.
13. An example of a mineral.
15. Protein is made of these.
16. What you gain by learning about nutrients.
19. A type of food high in complex carbohydrate.
20. Nutrient needed for healthy skin and insulation.
22. The body can live for only a few days without this.
23. A food high in added sugar.
24. A type of food with complete protein.
25. Nutrient that repairs body cells.
26. A kind of oil that has been turned into a solid fat.

Down

1. Pills, powders, or liquids that contain nutrients.
2. An example of a B vitamin.
3. An example of fat.
4. Type of carbohydrate found in starch.
5. An example of a saturated oil.
6. The process of breaking down food in the body.
11. Proteins that lack one or more of the essential amino acids.
12. The body's main source of energy.
14. Fats that are liquid at room temperature.
17. Nutrients that help other nutrients work properly.
18. Protein is needed to make these in the body. (2 words)
20. Plant material that does not break down during digestion.
21. A chemical the body needs to work properly.

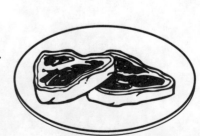

Continued on next page

Copyright © Glencoe/McGraw-Hill

Chapter 5: Puzzling Over Nutrients (*Continued*)

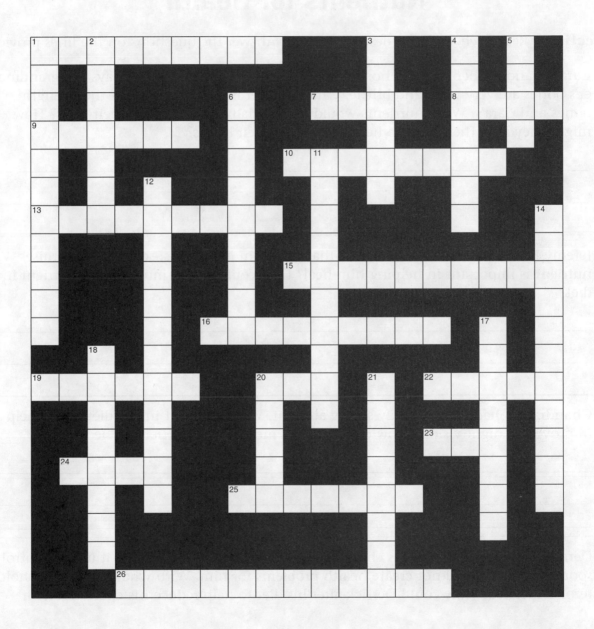

| CHAPTER **5** | | Text Pages 34-45 |

Meet the Nutrients

Nutrients for Health

Directions: Read each situation described below. Answer the questions on the lines provided.

1. Cara's grandmother is in the hospital with a broken hip. The doctor says her grandmother's bones are very weak and brittle. Cara's mother is concerned about the strength of her bones and Cara's. What nutrients would be especially important in their diets? How might they alter their diets to help strengthen their bones?

   _____

   _____

   _____

2. Jeremy had a skateboarding accident that gave him many cuts, scrapes, and bruises. What nutrient is important in helping him heal? How could he get more of this nutrient in his diet?

   _____

   _____

   _____

3. Chandra has had trouble lately seeing at night. What nutrient in her diet might help improve her night vision? How could she get more of the nutrient in her food?

   _____

   _____

   _____

4. Derrick has been told that his cholesterol is high for a teen. If he gets it under control soon, it probably will not create health problems for him. With what nutrient is cholesterol associated? How could Derrick alter his diet to help reduce his cholesterol?

   _____

   _____

   _____

Name _____ Date _____ Class Period _____

CHAPTER **6**

Energy and Calories

Study Guide

Directions: Answer the following questions on the lines provided.

1. Why are calories important in a healthy diet?

_____

_____

2. Which nutrients in food provide energy?

_____

_____

3. Why do different foods have different numbers of calories?

_____

_____

4. Why is serving size important in calculating calories?

_____

_____

_____

5. What percent of a healthy diet should be carbohydrate? Fat? Protein?

_____

_____

6. What is nutrient density? Why is it important?

_____

_____

_____

7. List two factors that help determine how many calories you need to eat each day.

_____

_____

Continued on next page

8. What is basal metabolic rate (BMR)?

_____

_____

9. Does everyone have the same BMR? Why or why not?

_____

_____

10. What is the relationship between calories used and level of physical activity?

_____

_____

11. Why is weight gain natural during the teen years?

_____

_____

12. List two ways you could increase your activity level.

_____

_____

_____

CHAPTER 6
Energy and Calories

Calorie Math

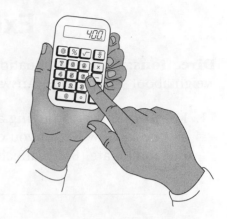

Directions: Read the following descriptions of food.
Refer to the chart on page 47 of the textbook. Do the
necessary calculation and write the answer on the lines
provided.

1. A serving of bagel chips contains 20 grams of carbohydrate, 3 grams of fat, and 3 grams
   of protein. How many calories would be in the serving of chips?

   _____

2. A hamburger has 445 calories. If you add a slice of cheese with 50 calories, how many
   calories would be in the cheeseburger?

   _____

3. A serving of cranberry oat cereal contains 200 calories per serving. Each serving contains
   three grams of fat. How many calories in the serving come from protein and carbohydrate?

   _____

4. A pizza contains 780 calories and serves two people. How many calories are in a serving?

   _____

5. A ½-cup serving of ice cream contains 140 calories. How many calories would be in a 3/4-
   cup serving?

   _____

6. A box mix of macaroni and cheese makes three one-cup servings. Each serving is 410
   calories. If a person ate half of the prepared mix, how many calories would that serving
   contain?

   _____

7. A ½-cup serving of prepared stuffing contains 170 total calories. The serving gets 134 calories from protein and carbohydrate. How many grams of fat are in a serving of the stuffing?

   _____

CHAPTER 6
Energy and Calories

Exercise and Calories

Directions: Read each situation described below. Assume all students in the situations below weigh about 140 pounds. Answer the questions on the lines provided.

1. Katrina has been studying all evening. She wonders if she burned any calories just sitting at a desk. How would you calculate how many calories she used? How would her basic metabolic rate (BMR) affect the answer?

_____

_____

_____

_____

_____

2. How many calories will Damon use if he runs fast for 30 minutes?

_____

3. How many calories will Dana use if she walks briskly for 10 minutes to warm up, then plays an hour of basketball?

_____

4. Louie has been cleaning his family's apartment and garage for the last two hours. He gets out two bagels to eat as a snack. He notices that the bagels each contain 150 calories. He wonders if he burned off more calories than that cleaning. Did he? Explain your answer.

_____

_____

5. Moira and her cousin have started riding their bikes after school. They ride for about 25 minutes on Tuesdays and Thursdays. Moira assumes she can have a high-calorie snack, such as chocolate cake, on those days, in addition to her regular meals and snacks. She assumes the exercise cancels out the chocolate cake calories. Is she correct?

_____

_____

6. Jett is starving after football practice. Explain why he is so hungry.

_____

_____

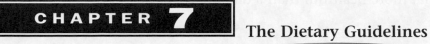

CHAPTER 7

The Dietary Guidelines

Study Guide

Directions: Answer the following questions on the lines provided.

1. What are food guides?

   _____

   _____

2. What are the Dietary Guidelines for Americans?

   _____

   _____

3. In using the Dietary Guidelines for Americans, what does the word "diet" mean?

   _____

   _____

4. To whom do the Dietary Guidelines for Americans apply?

   _____

   _____

5. Why should you eat a variety of foods?

   _____

   _____

6. How might a person's weight affect health?

   _____

   _____

7. Why do the Dietary Guidelines for Americans stress eating lots of grains, vegetables, and fruits?

   _____

   _____

   _____

Continued on next page

8. Why is a diet moderate in fat more healthful than a diet higher in fat?

_____

_____

9. Give two suggestions for reducing the amount of fat in your diet.

_____

_____

_____

10. Why is a diet high in sugar likely to be out of balance?

_____

_____

_____

11. What health problem is linked to eating too much sodium?

_____

_____

12. List one way to cut down on the amount of sodium you eat.

_____

_____

_____

CHAPTER 7

The Dietary Guidelines

Living the Guidelines

Directions: Read the situations described below. Answer each question on the lines provided.

1. Ross spends most of his time before and after school watching television or using his computer to surf the Internet or play computer games. He eats a balanced diet and watches how much fat, sugar, and salt he eats. Is Ross following the Dietary Guidelines? Explain your answer.

   _____

   _____

2. Noree loves burgers. Often she has one for lunch and another at dinner. Is Noree following the Dietary Guidelines? Explain your answer.

   _____

   _____

3. Pedro watches his diet carefully. He works out at least three times a week at the gym. He eats lots of legumes, vegetables, and fruits. He avoids fats and sugar. Is Pedro following the Dietary Guidelines? Explain your answer.

   _____

   _____

4. Kristin has a sweet tooth and she loves desserts. She usually has a sweet snack in the afternoon and at bedtime. Sometimes she eats dessert for breakfast! Is Kristin following the Dietary Guidelines? Explain your answer.

   _____

   _____

5. Drew never gains weight no matter what he eats. He is out for baseball, so he exercises every day during the season. Because he doesn't gain weight and exercises, he believes he can eat whatever he wants and have a healthy diet. Is this true? Explain your answer.

   _____

   _____

CHAPTER **7**

The Dietary Guidelines

Taking Action

Directions: Read each situation described below. Answer the question on the lines provided.

1. Dirk has just been told that he has high blood pressure. He needs to take action for the sake of his health. What Dietary Guideline would help Dirk improve his blood pressure? Why?

   _____

   _____

2. Jennifer has always been a picky eater. She only likes certain foods. She never tries anything new. How could Jennifer take action to use the Dietary Guidelines to improve her diet?

   _____

   _____

3. Demarco's father works at a desk job. He spends most of his evenings and weekends at the computer. Which Dietary Guideline could help improve his fitness?

   _____

   _____

4. Bailey loves French fries and chicken-fried steak. She would eat them every day if she could. If she did, would she be following the Dietary Guidelines? Explain your answer.

   _____

   _____

5. Timothy lost weight after he broke his jaw. He has decided to eat lots of desserts, especially pie and ice cream, to help him gain back the weight. Does his plan follow the Dietary Guidelines? Why or why not?

   _____

   _____

6. Ellie's family eats the same foods over and over. For instance, Monday is tuna casserole night. How could she take action to put more variety in the family diet?

   _____

   _____

CHAPTER 8

Text Pages 60-69

The Food Guide Pyramid

Study Guide

Directions: Answer the following questions on the lines provided.

1. What are two ways you can use the Food Guide Pyramid?

   _____

   _____

2. Which of the food groups on the Food Guide Pyramid is most important?

   _____

   _____

3. Why is the significance of the pyramid shape of the Food Guide Pyramid?

   _____

   _____

   _____

4. What characteristics are shared by the foods in the small section at the top of the Pyramid?

   _____

   _____

5. What do the small circles and triangles found throughout the Pyramid mean?

   _____

   _____

6. Why do you need to know Pyramid serving sizes?

   _____

   _____

7. How can you make healthful food choices when choosing foods from each food group?

   _____

   _____

Continued on next page

8. What are three grain products included in the Bread, Cereal, Rice, and Pasta Group?

_____

_____

9. Why should you eat a variety of vegetables? What nutrients can be found in foods from the Vegetable Group?

_____

_____

_____

10. Name a fruit that is high in vitamin C.

_____

11. Which Pyramid food group is a good source of calcium? How many servings from this group should teens have each day?

_____

12. Why are dry beans and peas an important part of the Meat, Poultry, Fish, Dry Beans, Eggs, and Nuts Group?

_____

_____

CHAPTER **8**

The Food Guide Pyramid

Food Groups and Nutrients

Directions: The five main food groups from the Food Guide Pyramid are shown below. Match the nutrients listed below to the food groups they come from. Write the letter of the food group(s) in the blank(s) to the left of each nutrient. Some nutrients are found in more than one food group, so blanks are given for each food group.

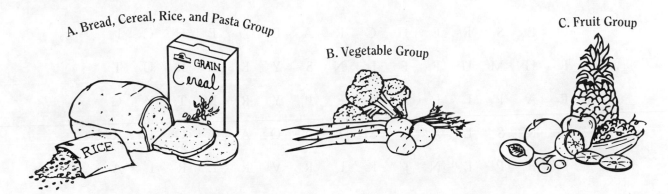

A. Bread, Cereal, Rice, and Pasta Group

B. Vegetable Group

C. Fruit Group

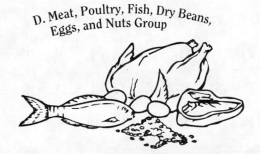

D. Meat, Poultry, Fish, Dry Beans, Eggs, and Nuts Group

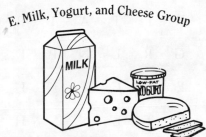

E. Milk, Yogurt, and Cheese Group

Nutrients

1. ____ Calcium

2. ____ ____ ____ Carbohydrate

3. ____ ____ B vitamins

4. ____ ____ ____ Fiber

5. ____ ____ Iron

6. ____ Magnesium

7. ____ Potassium

8. ____ ____ Protein

9. ____ ____ Beta-carotene

10. ____ ____ Vitamin C

11. ____ Zinc

Discovering Food and Nutrition Student Workbook **41**

Name _____ Date _____ Class Period _____

CHAPTER 8

The Food Guide Pyramid

Text Pages 60-69

Hidden Foods

Directions: Hidden in the puzzle below are 20 common foods. They may be listed forward, backward, horizontally, or vertically. Circle the foods, then decide in which food group they belong on the Food Guide Pyramid. Write the names of the foods in the blanks under the correct food group names.

```
O E S E E H C R A D D E H C I
F H M U F F I N S Y E K R U T
R A P P L E R F P Y R M T Y G
G M S L A E M T A O A K O L R
I B P E N J K I R V R L R I A
L U L T B T P E A R E I T N P
O R I T A T R U G O Y M I O E
C G R U N P F O U D K M L R F
C E H C A N I P S E U I L A R
O R T E N S H R I M P K A C U
R K S N A C E P U R T S S A I
B I B U T T E R M I L K C M T
```

Bread, Cereal, Rice, and Pasta Group	Vegetable Group	Fruit Group	Meat, Poultry, Fish, Dry Beans, Eggs, and Nuts Group	Milk, Yogurt, and Cheese Group

42 DISCOVERING FOOD AND NUTRITION Student Workbook

Copyright © Glencoe/McGraw-Hill

CHAPTER **9**

Your Daily Food Choices

Study Guide

Directions: Answer the following questions on the lines provided.

1. What kind of food choices would people who value good health be most likely to make?

_____

_____

2. How does technology affect food choices?

_____

_____

_____

3. What kinds of mass media can affect a person's food choices?

_____

_____

4. What skills can help you evaluate whether food and nutrition information is reliable?

_____

_____

5. List three reliable sources of food and nutrition information.

_____

_____

_____

6. How can you add variety to your diet?

_____

_____

7. What is a meal pattern? What meal pattern is most healthful?

_____

_____

_____

Continued on next page

8. What are three possible results of skipping meals?

_____

_____

_____

9. Why is breakfast the most important meal of the day? What might happen if you often skip breakfast?

_____

_____

_____

10. What are the advantages of eating meals at home?

_____

_____

11. What does it mean to be a vegetarian?

_____

_____

12. How do vegetarians get enough protein in their diets?

_____

_____

CHAPTER 9

Your Daily Food Choice

Is It True?

Directions: Read the following situations. On the lines provided, indicate if you think the information is true or false. Explain why you do or do not think it is believable.

1. A newspaper article says the Food and Drug Administration has approved a new medication that will benefit people who are seriously overweight.

   _____

   _____

2. A talk show host discusses one way that she controls her weight—by skipping breakfast.

   _____

   _____

3. Your friend's hairdresser says that vegetarians face a lot of health problems, because without meat their diets are inadequate.

   _____

   _____

4. The owner of the health food store promotes a powder to mix with juice that will restore good health to people with certain health problems.

   _____

   _____

5. An Internet website says it is all right to eat several small meals throughout the day instead of three official meals daily. The information is supplied by a registered dietitian and sponsored by a state university.

   _____

   _____

6. A new book features a weight-loss diet that allows you to eat as much food as you want, except no fruits or breads are allowed. The author has been promoting the plan on TV.

   _____

   _____

   _____

CHAPTER 9 Your Daily Food Choices

A Key to a Good Eating Plan

Directions: Complete this word scramble to identify the key to healthy food choices. The definition provides a clue for each word. Write the answer in the blanks provided, one letter per blank. Unscramble the circled letters to discover the word that belongs in the key.

1. __ __ __ __ __ ○ __ __   Something about you that influences the food choices you make.

2. __ __ ○ __ __ __ __ __ __ __ __   This is used to sell food products.

3. __ __ __ __ __ __ __ __ __ __ ○ __ __ __   What is needed to evaluate food claims. (2 words)

4. __ __ __ __ __ __ ○ __ __ __   A term that means avoiding extremes when you choose how much to eat.

5. __ __ __ __ __ __ __ ○ __ __   How often you eat snacks and meals during a day. (2 words)

6. __ __ ○ __ __ __   Besides meals, you probably eat these most days.

7. __ ○ __ __ __ __ __ __ __ __   The most important meal of the day.

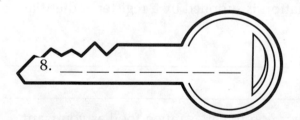

8. __ __ __ __ __ __ __   The key to satisfaction in making food choices.

Name _____ Date _____ Class Period _____

Study Guide

Directions: Answer the following questions on the lines provided.

1. Why is it important to make healthful food choices when eating out?

   _____

   _____

   _____

2. List two factors that affect people's choices of where to eat when they eat out.

   _____

3. How might a restaurant make nutrition information available to customers?

   _____

4. What does it mean when a restaurant has a special health symbol next to some menu items?

   _____

   _____

   _____

5. How can selecting a restaurant with a large menu help you make healthful food choices?

   _____

   _____

6. Give two suggestions for lowering the fat content of foods eaten in restaurants.

   _____

   _____

   _____

Continued on next page

7. Why is serving size a concern when eating out?

_____

_____

_____

8. When would it NOT be appropriate to ask a server to pack leftover food so you can take it home?

_____

_____

9. Why is portion control a special concern at salad bars and buffets?

_____

_____

10. What does "eating out" at home mean?

_____

_____

11. What food safety guidelines can help keep take-out or delivered food safe to eat?

_____

_____

12. Why should a take-out or delivered meal be placed in serving bowls or served on each person's plate?

_____

_____

CHAPTER 10   Eating Out

Top Choices

Directions: Read each situation described below. Answer the question on the lines provided.

1. You and a friend are trying to decide where to have lunch on a Saturday. One possibility is Connie's Cozy Cafe featuring a variety of fried foods. The other, Garden Deli, has a salad bar and a variety of cold meat and cheese sandwiches. Where would you be more likely to find low-fat choices? In making your lunch selection, what would you have to watch?

_____

_____

2. Chad's dinner comes with a choice of a potato or a vegetable. The orange juice he had at breakfast was his only serving from the fruit and vegetable group for the day. Tonight's choices are French fries, mashed potatoes and gravy, fresh green beans, and glazed carrots. Which should he choose? Why?

_____

_____

3. You have ordered a baked potato for lunch and are at the "Fixins" bar. Your choices are: butter, sour cream, chives, cheese sauce, grated cheese, chopped broccoli, crumbled bacon, taco sauce, and salsa. Which toppings would add the fewest calories to the potato? Which would add the most?

_____

_____

_____

4. Gabrielle is trying to decide what to order at a new restaurant: oven-baked cod, spaghetti with meat sauce, or zesty chili. She likes fish, but her family doesn't care for it. She wonders if the spaghetti would be as good as Grandma's. The chili sounds a little spicy. What do you think she should order?

_____

_____

| **CHAPTER 10** | | Text Pages 78-83 |

Eating Out

The All-You-Can-Eat Buffet

Directions: Read the situations described below. Answer each question on the lines provided.

Zachary and his grandfather are eating out at the All-You-Can-Eat Buffet, his grandfather's favorite restaurant. Zachary enjoys it too, piling his plate high, and returning several times to different buffet tables.

1. Zachary goes to the salad bar first. He sees lettuce and spinach salads, a variety of pasta and potato salads, and fresh fruit and vegetables. He wants to save some of his appetite for the buffet's hot foods. To ensure not getting too full, what would be wise choices from the salad bar?

   _____

   _____

2. After the salads, Zachary fills his plate with his favorites: fried fish fillets, Southern-fried chicken, deep-fried shrimp, French fries, and cheese sticks. Do you see a problem with the variety of his choices? Explain.

   _____

   _____

3. For dessert, Zachary piled his plate high with banana cake, blueberry pie, and a lemon bar. He told his grandfather that he'd chosen healthy desserts that all had fruit in them. What do you think of his reasoning? Explain your answer.

   _____

   _____

4. When Zachary and his grandfather leave the restaurant, they both complain about being too full and feeling uncomfortable. What advice would you give to help them prevent this feeling the next time?

   _____

   _____

Name _____ Date _____ Class Period _____

Study Guide

Directions: Answer the following questions on the lines provided.

1. What kinds of foods do babies eat?

   _____

   _____

2. What types of foods should not be fed to toddlers? Why?

   _____

   _____

3. Why do athletes usually need extra calories?

   _____

   _____

4. What is an eating disorder?

   _____

   _____

   _____

5. What do people with anorexia nervosa fear? Is this fear realistic? Explain.

   _____

   _____

6. Why is bulimia nervosa called a "binge and purge" disorder?

   _____

   _____

   _____

7. What is generally the cause of binge eating disorder?

   _____

   _____

Continued on next page

8. What should you do if you suspect a family member or friend has an eating disorder?

_____

_____

9. What causes food allergies?

_____

_____

10. Why can diabetes be a particularly dangerous disease?

_____

_____

11. Why is it important to read and follow directions when taking certain types of medicines?

_____

_____

_____

12. Why is good nutrition especially important during illness?

_____

_____

| CHAPTER **11** | Text Pages 84-89 |

Personalized Nutrition

Ask Morgan

Directions: Imagine that you write an advice column on diet and nutrition called "Ask Morgan." Read the following letters you have received and write your answers to the letters on the lines provided.

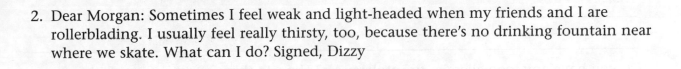

Dear Morgan,
I've got a problem
and I wanted to
know

1. Dear Morgan: I'm 15 years old and play basketball and soccer. I get hungry a lot so I usually eat about 10 times a day. My sister says I eat too much, but I don't gain weight. Am I overeating, like she says? Signed, Starving But Skinny

_____

_____

_____

2. Dear Morgan: Sometimes I feel weak and light-headed when my friends and I are rollerblading. I usually feel really thirsty, too, because there's no drinking fountain near where we skate. What can I do? Signed, Dizzy

_____

_____

_____

3. Dear Morgan: My doctor says I am developing a kind of diabetes. He told me I need to avoid any desserts or other foods with sugar. I love sweets. How am I going to stick to my diet? Signed, Sweet Tooth

_____

_____

_____

CHAPTER 11

Text Pages 84-89

Personalized Nutrition

A Personalized Plan

Directions: In personalizing nutrition, it is important to consider your unique needs and dietary conditions. Answer the following questions about yourself on the lines provided.

1. Have your food preferences changed since you were a young child? In what way? Do you expect that your nutritional needs will change as you become older?

   _____

   _____

   _____

2. Do you participate in sports or other physical activities such as dance? How does your participation (or lack of it) affect your nutritional needs?

   _____

   _____

3. What is your attitude toward food? Is it possible that you have an eating disorder?

   _____

   _____

4. Do you have any food allergies or intolerances? How do these affect your nutritional needs?

   _____

   _____

5. Do you take any medicines that would cause problems if eaten with certain foods? How do you adjust your diet to avoid these problems?

   _____

   _____

6. Summarize the way your diet needs to be adapted from the Pyramid Food Guide to take into account your personalized nutritional needs as you've described them in the above questions.

   _____

   _____

CHAPTER **12**

Shopping for Food

Study Guide

Directions: Answer the following questions on the lines provided.

1. List three things that affect the cost of food.

   _____

   _____

2. What factors should you consider in deciding how often to buy food?

   _____

   _____

3. What is the difference between a supermarket and a warehouse grocery store?

   _____

   _____

4. What is food processing? List three reasons foods are processed.

   _____

   _____

5. Why is planning meals the first step in making a shopping list?

   _____

   _____

   _____

6. List five pieces of information found on food labels.

   _____

   _____

   _____

Continued on next page

7. What is the UPC symbol used for?

_____

_____

8. The nutrition information on a food label is given for how many servings?

_____

9. Do you want a food with a high or low percent daily value of nutrients?

_____

_____

10. Does using a food before the date listed on the package mean the food will be of high quality? Why or why not?

_____

_____

11. What are three kinds of information to compare to get the best values when shopping for food?

_____

_____

12. What are five tips to help you buy good quality food?

_____

_____

_____

CHAPTER 12

Shopping for Food

What's the Unit Price?

Directions: Read the situations described below. Calculate the unit price of each product. Then tell which product you would recommend buying and explain why.

Laura is buying oatmeal. She serves it several days a week for breakfast and makes oatmeal cookies often. The grocery store has 18 oz. for $1.79 and 42 oz. for $2.98. Which should Laura buy?

1. Unit price:

    18 oz. _____   42 oz. _____

2. Recommendation: _____

3. Explanation: _____

    _____

    _____

Sergio is buying potatoes for his family. He finds a 5 lb. sack of potatoes for $1.99 and a 20 lb. sack for $4.99. Sergio has plenty of room to store the larger sack, but his family doesn't eat many potatoes. Which should Sergio buy?

4. Unit price:

    5 lb. sack_____   20 lb. sack_____

5. Recommendation: _____

6. Explanation: _____

    _____

    _____

Anvita is buying canola oil. A 24-ounce bottle costs $2.19. A 48-ounce bottle is $2.89. She is concerned that the larger bottle might be too tall to fit on the shelf where the oil is kept. The family does little baking, but has a stir-fry at least twice a week.

7. Unit price:

    24 oz. bottle_____   48 oz.bottle_____

8. Recommendations: _____

9. Explanation: _____

    _____

    _____

CHAPTER 12

Shopping for Food

Grocery Shopping

Directions: Listed below are clues that have to do with grocery shopping. Use each clue to fill in the blanks in the corresponding numbered item. The letters in the darker squares will spell a term that helps consumers buy food.

Clues

1. These depend on weather, time of year, packaging, and transportation. (2 words)

2. Put raw meat and poultry in this kind of bag.

3. Food may be displayed in cardboard boxes here.

4. This allows you to compare costs. (2 words)

5. If you make these wisely, you will get the most for your money.

6. These provide valuable information.

7. Some foods lose this if not brought home and stored immediately.

8. A kind of food buying to avoid.

9. This is often the least expensive brand.

10. Avoid this kind of container when buying food.

Name _____ Date _____ Class Period _____

CHAPTER 13 Using Kitchen Appliances

Study Guide

Directions: Answer the following questions on the lines provided.

1. What is the difference between large and small appliances?

   _____

   _____

   _____

2. How should the freezer section of a one-door refrigerator be used? Why?

   _____

   _____

   _____

3. Why should the wire shelves of a refrigerator or freezer be left uncovered?

   _____

   _____

4. What happens when frost builds up in the freezer? What can be done about it?

   _____

   _____

   _____

5. List and describe the three parts of a range.

   _____

   _____

   _____

6. Describe how food is cooked in the microwave.

   _____

   _____

   _____

Continued on next page

7. How can you avoid wasting heat when using the cooktop of the range?

_____

_____

8. Why should you adjust the oven racks before turning on heat?

_____

_____

9. What are the main advantages of using small appliances?

_____

_____

10. What is the difference between a toaster and a toaster oven?

_____

_____

11. For what food preparation jobs could you use a blender?

_____

_____

12. What does it mean when an appliance is labeled "immersible"?

_____

_____

CHAPTER 13

Using Kitchen Appliances

Identifying Small Appliances

Directions: Several small appliances are pictured below. The names of these appliances are given in scrambled form. Unscramble each word and write it in the blank above the appliance it names.

xrmei	tcieeclr tleksil	rasttoe	aosrett vnoe

wlos orckoe	dofo sropscroe	dreenlb

1. _____

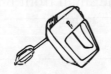

2. _____

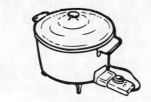

3. _____

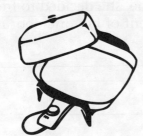

4. _____

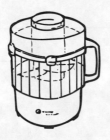

5. _____

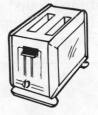

6. _____

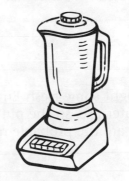

7. _____

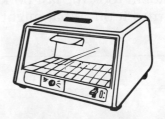

CHAPTER 13

Using Kitchen Appliances

What Might Happen?

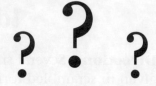

Directions: Read the situations described below. Then answer each item as directed.

1. Malcolm's family has a new convection oven. Malcolm prepares a cake mix and places the pan in the new oven for 35 minutes, just as he would have with their conventional oven. What might happen?

   _____

   _____

2. Natalie is warming soup in a large pan for lunch. She turned on the small front burner of the range to heat the soup. What could be the consequences of her actions

   _____

   _____

3. Shane wanted to check on the casserole he was baking in the oven, so he leaned his face close to the oven door and opened it a crack to peek at the casserole. What could be the consequences of his actions?

   _____

   _____

4. Briana bought some fresh English muffins. When she got home, she decided to freeze them for later use, so she put them in the freezing compartment of her one-door refrigerator. What are the probable results of her action?

   _____

   _____

5. When Robin took the last pork chop out of the electric skillet, she unplugged the skillet, then turned it off. What might have happened?

   _____

   _____

CHAPTER **14**
Know Your Equipment

Study Guide

Directions: Answer the following questions on the lines provided.

1. What is the advantage of using special kitchen equipment when you prepare food?

   _____

   _____

2. Why should coffee cups and spoons used on the table not be used for measuring ingredients for cooking?

   _____

   _____

3. Why should knives be kept properly sharpened?

   _____

   _____

4. What is the purpose of a cutting board?

   _____

   _____

5. What foods might you choose to cut with kitchen shears rather than a knife?

   _____

   _____

6. What kind of tools should be used with pans with a nonstick finish? Why?

   _____

   _____

7. What kind of tool would be useful in removing peas from the liquid in which they were canned?

   _____

   _____

Continued on next page

8. What is the difference between an oven-proof thermometer and an instant-read thermometer? What are they used for?

_____

_____

_____

_____

9. List the various materials from which cookware can be made. Where can each be used?

_____

_____

_____

_____

10. What is the difference between a saucepan and a pot?

_____

_____

11. What is a casserole used for?

_____

_____

12. Why do baking pans come in a wide variety of shapes and sizes? Give examples.

_____

_____

_____

_____

Text Pages 108-115

CHAPTER 14
Know Your Equipment

Kitchen Equipment I.D.

Directions: Match each equipment name below with the correct sketch of the equipment. Write the letter of the equipment name in the blank above each pictured item. Do not use any name more than once. Some names will not be used.

A. Chef's knife	B. Colander	C. Cutting board
D. Dry measuring cups	E. Grater	F. Kitchen shears
G. Ladle	H. Liquid measuring cup	I. Pastry blender
J. Peeler	K. Rolling pin	L. Rotary beater
M. Rubber scraper	N. Serrated knife	O. Sifter
P. Spatula	Q. Tongs	R. Wire cooling rack

____1. ____2. ____3. ____4.

____5. ____6. ____7. ____8.

____9. ____10. ____11. ____12.

____13. ____14. ____15. ____16.

CHAPTER 14

Know Your Equipment

What Equipment is Needed?

Directions: Read the situations described below. List the equipment needed on the lines provided.

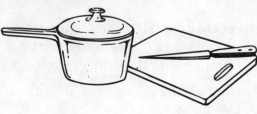

1. Francessca is making a loaf of applesauce bread. The recipe includes sifted flour, milk, baking soda, applesauce, a beaten egg, and spices. What equipment does Francessca need to make and bake this recipe?

   _____

   _____

   _____

   _____

2. David is making a tossed salad for supper. He's using lettuce, grated carrots, sliced celery and cucumbers, and shredded cheddar cheese. What equipment does he need to make this salad?

   _____

   _____

   _____

   _____

3. Kaitlin is making sauce to serve over spaghetti. The sauce recipe calls for ground beef, chopped onions and green peppers, sliced celery, tomato sauce, and several spices. What equipment will Kaitlin need to make the spaghetti and sauce?

   _____

   _____

   _____

   _____

CHAPTER 15

Reading Recipes

Study Guide

Directions: Answer the following questions on the lines provided.

1. What basic information should a recipe provide so it can be made successfully?

   _____

   _____

2. What is the yield of a recipe?

   _____

   _____

3. In making what type of products should you follow the recipe exactly for best results?

   _____

   _____

4. What is a substitution chart?

   _____

   _____

5. What are the similarities and differences between chopping and mincing?

   _____

   _____

   _____

   _____

6. What is the difference between stirring and beating a mixture?

   _____

   _____

   _____

Continued on next page

7. When a cookie recipe says to cream sugar and shortening, what does it mean?

_____

_____

8. Explain how to fold in ingredients.

_____

_____

_____

_____

9. Why should an appliance like an oven be preheated?

_____

_____

10. Explain the different ways food can be browned. How do you know which method to choose?

_____

_____

11. What type of food product should be used to grease a pan?

_____

_____

12. What is the purpose of a garnish?

_____

_____

CHAPTER 15

Reading Recipes

Understanding the Recipe

Directions: Read the recipe and answer the questions below on the lines provided.

One-Dish Dinner

Customary	Ingredients
1 lb.	Ground Beef
1	Onion, chopped
1 10¾ oz. can	Condensed tomato soup
1 16 oz. can	Green beans, drained
¼ tsp.	Ground pepper
1½ cup	Mashed potatoes
⅓ cup	Shredded cheddar cheese

Yield: 4 servings

Pan: 12-inch skillet
2-quart casserole dish

Directions

1. **Preheat** oven to 350°F.
2. **Crumble** ground beef in skillet. Add onion and cook until browned.
3. **Spoon** off excess fat.
4. **Add** tomato soup, green beans, and pepper.
5. **Simmer** five minutes.
6. **Grease** casserole dish. Pour meat mixture into casserole.
7. **Drop** potatoes in mounds onto hot meat mixture.
8. **Sprinkle** with shredded cheese.
9. **Bake** for 20 minutes.

---

1. What ingredients are used to make this recipe?_____

_____

2. What size measuring cups and spoons are needed to make this recipe?_____

_____

3. What tools are needed to chop the onion?_____

4. What will the onion be like after it is chopped? _____

_____

5. What does it mean to drain the green beans? What tool(s) could be used to drain them?

_____

6. What tool would you use to shred the cheese? _____

7. How many people will this recipe serve?_____

CHAPTER **15**

Reading Recipes

Magic Terms Square

Directions: Find the term that best fits each description. Write the number of the correct term in the space in the lettered square. If all your answers are correct, the total of the numbers, or the "Magic Number," will be the same in each row across and down. Write the Magic Number in the space provided.

Terms

1. baste	11. mince
2. beat	12. pare
3. boil	13. preheat
4. chill	14. puree
5. cream	15. shred
6. cube	16. slice
7. cut in	17. stir
8. drain	18. toss
9. fold in	19. whip
10. garnish	

A	B	C	D
E	F	G	H
I	J	K	L
M	N	O	P

The Magic Number is _____.

Descriptions

A. To mix with a rotary beater or electric mixer.

B. To mix shortening and flour with a pastry blender.

C. To tumble a mixture very lightly with a spoon and fork.

D. To cut a thin layer of peel from fruits or vegetables.

E. To remove excess liquid from a food.

F. To combine shortening and sugar until soft and smooth.

G. To chop food until the pieces are as small as possible.

H. To cut food into long, thin pieces.

I. To turn on an oven ahead of time.

J. To mix using a circular or figure eight motion.

K. To cut into pieces that are ½-inch square or larger.

L. To heat a liquid until bubbles constantly rise to the surface and break.

M. To cut into thin, flat pieces.

N. To decorate a food or dish with a small, colorful food.

O. To refrigerate food until it is cold.

P. To gently combine two mixtures.

Name _____ Date _____ Class Period _____

CHAPTER 16 Recipe Math

Study Guide

Directions: Answer the following questions on the lines provided.

1. Why are math skills needed in preparing food?

_____

_____

2. Who uses the U.S. standard or customary system of measurement? The metric system?

_____

_____

3. Why is it helpful to know equivalents?

_____

_____

4. What kitchen equipment is used to measure volume?

_____

_____

5. What measurements of weight are typically used in food preparation?

_____

_____

6. Why can use of the term "ounces" be confusing in food preparation?

_____

_____

7. What is the difference between yield and desired yield?

_____

_____

8. What is the formula for increasing or decreasing a recipe?

_____

_____

Continued on next page

9. How does the cook use the magic number from the yield formula?

_____

_____

_____

10. Why may you need to convert or use an equivalent measure when adjusting a recipe?

_____

_____

11. Explain how rounding off ingredient measures could affect a stew and a cake.

_____

_____

_____

12. How should pan size be adjusted when a recipe is decreased?

_____

_____

Recipe Math

Abbreviating Terms

Directions: Match each measuring term in the left column with the correct abbreviation from the right column. Write the letter of the abbreviation in the space provided. Do not use any abbreviation more than once. Some abbreviations will not be used.

Measuring Terms	Abbreviation
____ 1. Celsius	A. kg
____ 2. Centimeter	B. m
____ 3. Cup	C. pd.
____ 4. Gallon	D. lb.
____ 5. Gram	E. C
____ 6. Inch	F. L
____ 7. Kilogram	G. oz.
____ 8. Liter	H. g
____ 9. Milliliter	I. tsp.
____ 10. Millimeter	J. qt.
____ 11. Ounce	K. cm
____ 12. Pint	L. pt.
____ 13. Pound	M. Tbsp.
____ 14. Quart	N. c.
____ 15. Tablespoon	O. gal.
____ 16. Teaspoon	P. mL
	Q. in.
	R. mm

Looking at Equivalents

Directions: Look at the two measurement terms listed in the lenses of the glasses below and write the equivalent measure in the space provided.

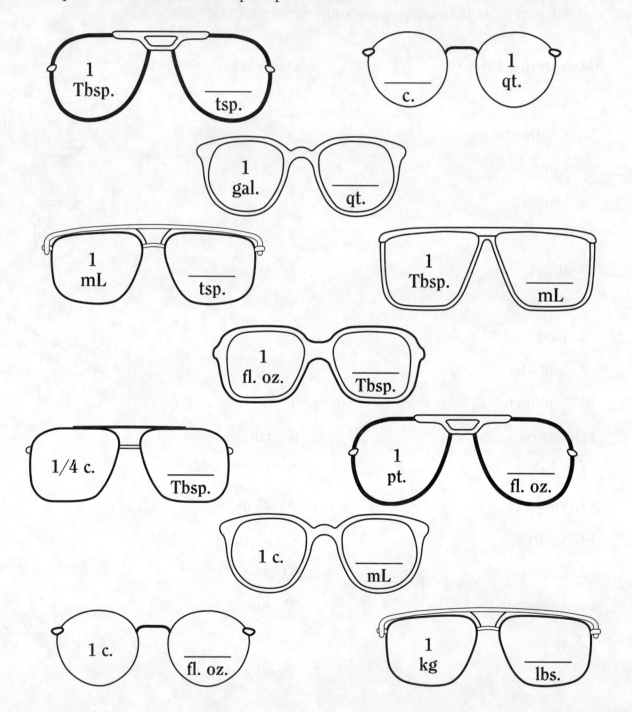

1 Tbsp. _____ tsp.

_____ c. 1 qt.

1 gal. _____ qt.

1 mL _____ tsp.

1 Tbsp. _____ mL

1 fl. oz. _____ Tbsp.

1/4 c. _____ Tbsp.

1 pt. _____ fl. oz.

1 c. _____ mL

1 c. _____ fl. oz.

1 kg _____ lbs.

CHAPTER 17
Basic Measuring Methods

Study Guide

Directions: Answer the following questions on the lines provided.

1. Why is measuring ingredients accurately important in preparing food?

   _____

   _____

2. What are two specific ingredients that are measured using dry measuring cups and measuring spoons?

   _____

   _____

3. How do you use a spatula when measuring dry ingredients?

   _____

   _____

4. Why should a measuring cup or spoon be held over waxed paper or the ingredient container while you are measuring?

   _____

   _____

   _____

5. What special steps are needed when measuring granulated sugar?

   _____

   _____

6. How do you sift flour? What does sifting do to the flour?

   _____

   _____

7. What types of flours are not sifted?

   _____

Continued on next page

8. Why should a liquid measuring cup be used to measure liquids?

_____

_____

9. Why would you oil a measuring cup before measuring corn syrup?

_____

_____

10. Why should a liquid measuring cup be on a flat surface while measuring?

_____

_____

11. Describe how to check the level of liquid in a measuring cup. Why is this necessary?

_____

_____

_____

12. What tools and equipment are needed to do the dry measuring cup method of measuring shortening?

_____

_____

CHAPTER **17** Basic Measuring Methods

How Do You Measure . . .?

Directions: The ingredients shown below are measured with a variety of measuring methods. Match each ingredient with two or more of the measuring methods listed below. Write the letter of the appropriate measuring methods in the blanks under the ingredients. There is one blank for each measuring method.

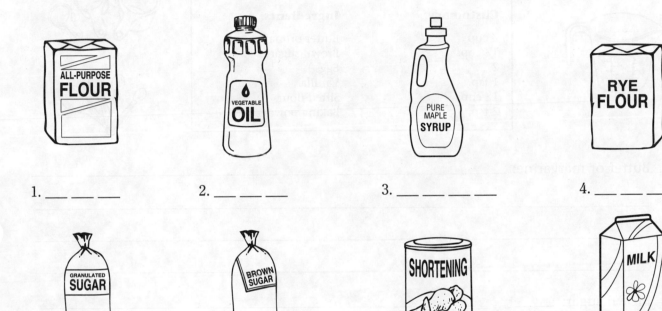

1. ___ ___ ___   2. ___ ___ ___   3. ___ ___ ___ ___   4. ___ ___ ___

5. ___ ___ ___   6. ___ ___ ___   7. ___ ___ ___   8. ___ ___ ___

Measuring Methods

A. Use a dry measuring cup.

B. Use a liquid measuring cup.

C. May need sifting (or straining) before use.

D. Check measurement at eye level.

E. Pack firmly in cup.

F. Level with a straight edge.

G. Never sift.

H. Be sure to work out air bubbles.

I. Measure on a flat surface.

J. Grease or oil cup before measuring.

Name _____ Date _____ Class Period _____

Recipe Measuring

Directions: Given below is the ingredient list for a recipe of Butterscotch Bars. On the lines below, explain what type and size of cups or spoons should be used and how the listed ingredient should be measured.

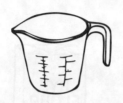

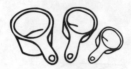

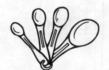

Butterscotch Bars

Customary	Ingredients
½ cup	Butter or margarine
1½ cups	Brown sugar
2	Eggs
1 tsp.	Vanilla
1½ cups	Sifted flour
2 tsp.	Baking powder

1. Butter or margarine: _____

_____

_____

_____

2. Brown sugar: _____

_____

_____

3. Vanilla: _____

_____

_____

4. Sifted flour: _____

_____

_____

5. Baking powder: _____

_____

_____

CHAPTER 18
Basic Cooking Terms

Study Guide

Directions: Answer the following questions on the lines provided.

1. Why is it important to understand the three basic methods of cooking food?

   _____

   _____

2. What does it mean to cook a food in dry heat?

   _____

   _____

3. What is the difference between baking and roasting?

   _____

   _____

4. How do you control how fast food cooks when it is broiled?

   _____

   _____

5. Describe how to panbroil a hamburger.

   _____

   _____

6. What does it mean to cook a food in moist heat?

   _____

   _____

Continued on next page

7. What is a common way to steam a food?

_____

_____

_____

8. What does it mean to fry a food?

_____

_____

9. What is the main difference between deep-fat frying and panfrying?

_____

_____

_____

10. How are foods prepared for sautéing?

_____

_____

11. What two basic cooking methods are involved in stir-frying?

_____

_____

12. Identify three ways that nutrients can be lost when food is prepared.

_____

_____

CHAPTER 18   Basic Cooking Terms

Hidden Cooking Terms

Directions: Hidden in the puzzle below are 13 cooking terms. The terms may appear forward, backward, horizontally, or vertically. Circle each term in the puzzle. Decide which type of cooking method each term is and write it in the appropriate space in the chart below.

```
G  N  I  Y  R  F  H  C  N  E  R  F  S
N  R  B  H  C  G  L  R  F  S  T  M  M
I  N  S  O  G  N  I  S  I  A  R  B  B
V  T  T  R  B  I  W  B  S  B  P  I  R
A  Y  E  V  O  Y  D  O  E  A  A  N  O
W  P  A  N  B  R  O  I  L  I  N  G  I
O  G  M  N  S  F  D  L  I  N  F  N  L
R  N  I  G  J  R  E  I  K  F  R  I  I
C  I  N  G  I  I  P  N  Z  F  Y  E  N
I  K  G  O  T  T  O  G  S  M  I  T  G
M  A  R  O  A  S  T  I  N  G  N  U  I
A  B  A  I  N  G  A  I  C  N  G  A  S
G  E  T  G  N  I  R  E  M  M  I  S  P
```

Dry Heat	Moist Heat	Frying	Combination

Discovering Food and Nutrition Student Workbook

Name _____ Date _____ Class Period _____

Predicting Consequences

Directions: Given below are situations involving foods and different cooking methods. Read each item and predict the consequences of the action(s) taken.

1. Katie wants to braise a pot roast with some vegetables. To save time she skips browning the meat first. Instead she starts it in liquid with the carrots and potatoes that she has cut in small pieces. What could be the consequences of her actions?

   _____

   _____

2. Jon is broiling chicken for dinner. He doesn't like to wash the broiler pan so he lines the grid with aluminum foil. What will be the consequences of his action?

   _____

   _____

3. Kelly is broiling a hamburger. Because it is thick and she wants it well done, she puts it close to the heating element. What will be the consequences of her action?

   _____

   _____

4. Dylan is simmering potatoes for potato salad. He is in a hurry, so he turns up the heat until the potatoes are boiling vigorously. What will be the consequences of his action?

   _____

   _____

5. Rashida is steaming broccoli. She puts the steamer basket in the pan, but doesn't cover the pan as the broccoli cooks. What will be the consequences of her action?

   _____

   _____

6. Whitney is making scrambled eggs for breakfast. She melts the butter in a small skillet over high heat and then adds the eggs to cook. What will be the consequences of her action?

   _____

   _____

Copyright © Glencoe/McGraw-Hill

CHAPTER 19

Microwave Techniques

Study Guide

Directions: Answer the following questions on the lines provided.

1. How can using a microwave oven help you save time?

   _____

   _____

2. What produces the heat that cooks food in a microwave oven?

   _____

   _____

3. What is the relationship between the cooking power of a microwave oven and its cooking speed?

   _____

   _____

4. When food is not uniform in size and shape, how should it be arranged for microwaving?

   _____

   _____

5. How would you decide whether to use an upside down plate or waxed paper to cover a dish in the microwave?

   _____

   _____

   _____

6. What procedure should be used to prevent overcooking microwaved foods?

   _____

   _____

   _____

Continued on next page

7. What is the result of having a microwave with a "hot spot"?

_____

_____

8. What can you do to help food cook evenly in a microwave?

_____

_____

9. What is the purpose of standing time?

_____

_____

10. Why should you use potholders to handle containers of microwaved foods?

_____

_____

11. How should whole foods, such as potatoes, be prepared to keep them from bursting when "baking" them in the microwave?

_____

_____

12. Why should spills and splatters in the microwave be wiped up immediately?

_____

_____

CHAPTER 19 Microwave Techniques

The Microwave File

Directions: The numbers beneath the answer blanks below correspond to the numbers on the drawers of the filing cabinet. Find the file drawer that corresponds with the number below the blank. Then determine which of the letters on the file drawer you need to spell the correct word. Write that letter in the appropriate space. If you think you know the term from the clue alone, use the file drawer numbers to check your accuracy.

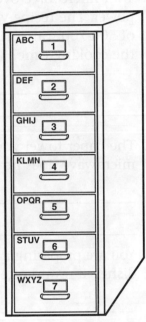

1. This is a major advantage of cooking with a microwave.

$\overline{}\ \overline{}\ \overline{}\ \overline{}\ \overline{}$ $\overline{}\ \overline{}\ \overline{}\ \overline{}$
   6 1 6 2 6   6 3 4 2

2. A type of food often made especially for microwave cooking.

$\overline{}\ \overline{}\ \overline{}\ \overline{}\ \overline{}\ \overline{}\ \overline{}\ \overline{}\ \overline{}\ \overline{}\ \overline{}$
   1 5 4 6 2 4 3 2 4 1 2

3. What food molecules do when penetrated by microwaves.

$\overline{}\ \overline{}\ \overline{}\ \overline{}\ \overline{}\ \overline{}\ \overline{}$
   6 3 1 5 1 6 2

4. Materials used in the microwave should have this label.

$\overline{}\ \overline{}\ \overline{}\ \overline{}\ \overline{}\ \overline{}\ \overline{}\ \overline{}\ \overline{}$ - $\overline{}\ \overline{}\ \overline{}\ \overline{}$
   4 3 1 5 5 7 1 6 2   6 1 2 2

5. This material should be used in the microwave as recommended in the owner's manual.

$\overline{}\ \overline{}\ \overline{}\ \overline{}\ \overline{}\ \overline{}\ \overline{}$ $\overline{}\ \overline{}\ \overline{}\ \overline{}$
   1 4 6 4 3 4 6 4   2 5 3 4

6. Food cooked in the microwave should be in this kind of pieces.

$\overline{}\ \overline{}\ \overline{}\ \overline{}\ \overline{}\ \overline{}\ \overline{}$
   6 4 3 2 5 5 4

7. Use this to cover food when microwaving if you want to hold in moisture.

$\overline{}\ \overline{}\ \overline{}\ \overline{}\ \overline{}\ \overline{}$ - $\overline{}\ \overline{}\ \overline{}\ \overline{}$ $\overline{}\ \overline{}\ \overline{}\ \overline{}\ \overline{}$
   6 5 6 3 2 2   2 5 7 4   5 4 1 6 2

8. This action will help food heat evenly in the microwave.

$\overline{}\ \overline{}\ \overline{}\ \overline{}\ \overline{}\ \overline{}$ $\overline{}\ \overline{}\ \overline{}\ \overline{}$
   5 5 6 1 6 2   2 3 6 3

Discovering Food and Nutrition Student Workbook **85**

Name _____ Date _____ Class Period _____

Using the Microwave

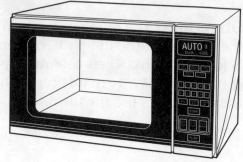

Directions: Read each situation described below.
Answer the question on the lines provided.

1. Your microwave oven has 900 watts of cooking
   power. The recipe you are using calls for an oven
   of 500-700 watts. How would you need to adjust
   the cooking time? Why?

   _____

   _____

2. The paper towel you have wrapped around the hotdog you are ready to heat in the
   microwave does not say "microwave-safe." Should you use it anyway? Why or why not?

   _____

   _____

3. You are preparing a casserole to cook in the microwave. You have two glass casserole
   dishes: a round one and a square one. Which should you choose? Why?

   _____

   _____

4. You want to heat a bun for your sandwich in the microwave. The last time you heated a
   bun, it ended up being hard as a rock. How can this be prevented?

   _____

   _____

5. Your microwave has "hot spots." How might you move potatoes to be sure they are thoroughly baked in the microwave?

   _____

   _____

CHAPTER 20

Safety in the Kitchen

Study Guide

Directions: Answer the following questions on the lines provided.

1. What causes accidents in the kitchen?

   _____

   _____

2. What are the most common accidents that occur in the kitchen?

   _____

   _____

3. Why should knives be washed separately from other dishes?

   _____

   _____

   _____

4. How should tiny pieces of broken glass be picked up?

   _____

   _____

5. Why should electrical cords be kept away from a sink?

   _____

   _____

6. Explain how to disconnect an appliance from the electrical outlet.

   _____

   _____

   _____

7. What does flammable mean? How should flammable items be handled?

   _____

   _____

   _____

Continued on next page

8. What is one possible result of using a wet potholder on a hot pan?

_____

_____

9. What common household products can be used to smother a grease fire? How do they work?

_____

_____

10. What can happen if a rug does not have a nonskid backing?

_____

_____

11. What are four ways poisons can enter the body? What should you do if someone is poisoned? Why?

_____

_____

_____

_____

12. Why should cleaning supplies not be kept in the same cabinets with foods?

_____

_____

CHAPTER **20**

Safety in the Kitchen

Seven Safety Errors

Directions: Read the scenario below. In the chart, write seven safety errors that Claire made, the type of accident that could have been caused, and what she should have done instead.

Claire was making tacos for supper. She needed the largest skillet for the taco meat, so she climbed on a kitchen chair to reach it. While the meat was browning, she covered it. Then she checked its progress by tipping the cover toward her to look at the meat. Then Claire drained the grease from the browned meat. She spilled some of the grease on the floor, but was in too much of a hurry to wipe it up. Claire had spilled the grease because the skillet handle was loose. She used a utility knife to tighten the loose screw on the handle. Claire started preparing the other taco ingredients. She opened a can of black olives about halfway, then bent back the lid and removed the olives for slicing. She chopped the onions and let-tuce. Then she preheated the oven to warm the taco shells. As she reached for the grater for the cheese, the knife started to fall off the counter. Claire tried to catch it, but it bounced off her shoe. Luckily she was wearing leather shoes. Thinking the oven wouldn't be very hot yet, Claire opened the oven door and pulled the rack out with her right hand.

Safety Error	Type of Accident	What Should Claire Have Done?
1.		
2.		
3.		
4.		
5.		
6.		
7.		

CHAPTER 20

Safety in the Kitchen

What's the Word?

Directions: The purpose of kitchen safety is to avoid the word inside the dark lines below. To discover what it is, read each clue below. Write the word or words that fit the clue on the corresponding line of the puzzle, one letter in each box.

1.
2.
3.
4.
5.
6.
7.
8.

Clues

1. A material that burns easily.

2. This can cause severe shocks and burns.

3. The kind of cabinet where household chemicals should be stored in a home with children.

4. Injury that can result from using dangerous chemicals.

5. Use this to reach items on high shelves.

6. One cause of many kitchen burns.

7. The kind of backing a rug used in the kitchen should have.

8. What grease can do if water is put on a grease fire.

9. The word is _____.

CHAPTER 21

Keeping Food Safe to Eat

Study Guide

Directions: Answer the following questions on the lines provided.

1. Identify three examples of harmful bacteria that cause foodborne illness.

   _____

   _____

   _____

2. What conditions are needed for bacteria to multiply?

   _____

   _____

3. How can you prevent food-borne illness when you work with food?

   _____

   _____

4. Describe the procedure for a thorough hand washing. Explain why you should wash your hands even if you are wearing gloves.

   _____

   _____

   _____

   _____

   _____

5. What guideline should you use to keep from spreading bacteria when you set the table?

   _____

   _____

   _____

6. How should a cutting board be cleaned? Why?

   _____

   _____

Continued on next page

7. Can the same towel be used as a hand towel and to dry dishes in the kitchen? Explain your answer.

_____

_____

8. Why should food not be thawed at room temperature?

_____

_____

9. How should you handle leftover hot food after a meal?

_____

_____

10. Why should the inside temperature of a refrigerator be between 32°F and 40°F?

_____

_____

11. How should bulk foods be stored? Why?

_____

_____

12. What are signs that a food may be spoiled?

_____

_____

CHAPTER **21**

Keeping Food Safe to Eat

Priority Storage

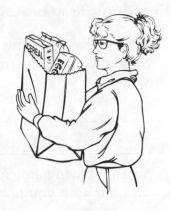

Directions: Read the case example described below. Then answer the questions on the lines provided.

The phone is ringing as Brittany arrives home from the supermarket. Her neighbor needs her to babysit immediately so she can take the baby to the doctor. Brittany has two bags of groceries to put away, but now has only a moment before she needs to hurry next door. The food in the bags includes: 2 fresh tomatoes, a head of cabbage, a box of macaroni, a bag of marshmallows, a carton of milk, three cans of soup, a carton of ice cream, fresh pears, a can of frozen grape juice, a package of ground beef, a box of frozen green beans, a carton of eggs, a carton of yogurt, a box mix for a cake, American cheese slices, and a box of breakfast cereal.

1. Which foods should Brittany put away before going to babysit? Where should these foods be stored?

   _____

   _____

   _____

   _____

2. Imagine that Brittany returns home two hours later and discovers that she forgot to put the ground beef away. What should she do? Why?

   _____

   _____

   _____

3. Explain where Brittany should store the foods remaining in the grocery bags.

   _____

   _____

   _____

4. Brittany is hungry and would like to heat something for supper. In the refrigerator, there is some chili left from either four or five days earlier. Would you recommend that she eat the chili? Explain.

   _____

   _____

CHAPTER 21

Keeping Food Safe to Eat

What Would You Do?

Directions: Read each situation described below. Answer the question on the lines provided.

1. A friend says you can eat raw foods after they are frozen because freezing kills bacteria. Should you eat the frozen uncooked chocolate chip cookie dough she offers you? Why or why not?

_____

_____

2. You are having a picnic on a cool spring day. Your fried chicken has been out for about an hour. Can you take home the leftovers and use them tomorrow? Explain your answer.

_____

_____

3. A package of ground beef that is thawing in the refrigerator has dripped liquid on a bowl of leftover pudding. Would you eat the pudding? Explain your answer.

_____

_____

4. Your family wants to have grilled chicken after your sister's softball game. Since everybody will be very hungry by then, someone suggests partially baking the chicken before the game, refrigerating it, and then finishing it on the grill. Is this a good way to save time? Why or why not?

_____

_____

5. You are making a stir-fry that contains strips of beef, chopped onions, broccoli, and chopped peanuts. You only have one cutting board. In what order would you do the jobs that require the cutting board? Explain your answer.

_____

_____

_____

CHAPTER 22 Getting Organized

Study Guide

Directions: Answer the following questions on the lines provided.

1. What is the first step in getting organized in the kitchen?

   _____

   _____

2. What resources can you draw upon in food preparation?

   _____

   _____

3. What is a work plan? How is one used in food preparation?

   _____

   _____

4. Why is pre-preparation an important step in preparing a recipe?

   _____

   _____

5. How do you know when to start food preparation?

   _____

   _____

6. What is benefit of gathering all ingredients and equipment first?

   _____

   _____

7. How does dovetailing benefit you when you are preparing food?

   _____

   _____

Continued on next page

8. Why should dishes and equipment be put away as soon as they are dry?

_____

_____

9. Why is the time schedule especially important in a foods lab?

_____

_____

10. Give three suggestions for promoting teamwork in the foods lab.

_____

_____

_____

11. What does it mean to evaluate food?

_____

_____

12. How can teamwork be evaluated?

_____

_____

_____

Name _____ Date _____ Class Period _____

CHAPTER 22

Getting Organized

Planning Ahead

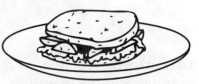

Directions: Read the recipe below. Then answer the questions on the lines provided.

Grilled Apple-Cheese Sandwiches	
Customary	**Ingredients**
1 cup	Sharp cheddar cheese, grated
1 cup	Apple, finely chopped
½ cup	Stuffed green olives, minced
⅓ cup	Mayonnaise
8 slices	Whole-wheat bread
¼ cup	Butter or margarine

Yield: 4 sandwiches

Pan: Nonstick griddle

Directions

1. **Combine** cheese, apple, olives, and mayonnaise in mixing bowl.
2. **Spread** mixture on four slices of bread.
3. **Top** with the other four slices of bread.
4. **Spread** butter or margarine on both outer sides of sandwiches.
5. **Heat** griddle over medium heat until a drop of water sizzles when splashed on the griddle.
6. **Grill** sandwiches for 2 to 3 minutes.
7. **Turn** over and grill 2 to 3 more minutes until bread is golden brown and cheese is melted.
8. **Serve** immediately.

1. List three pre-preparation tasks for this recipe and the equipment needed to complete them.

_____

_____

_____

2. Estimate how long (A) pre-preparation, (B) preparation, and (C) cooking time will take.

(A) _____ (B) _____ (C) _____

3. How long do you estimate this recipe will take to prepare? _____

4. When should you start cooking to have the sandwiches ready to eat at 6:30 p.m.?

_____

_____

5. Which two steps listed in the directions could be dovetailed? Explain. _____

_____

_____

CHAPTER 22
Getting Organized

Text Pages 172-179

Cook's Code

Directions: The answers to the following questions from the chapter are in code. Use the example and the questions to break the code. Then decode the mystery message in number 10.

Example: K I T C H E N   C O D E
          G E P Y D A J   Y K Z A

1. _ _ _ _ _ _ _ _ _
    A M Q E L I A J P

    What is a resource needed for food preparation?

2. _ _ _ _   _ _ _ _
    S K N G   L H W J

    What is a list of the jobs to be done in food preparation?

3. _ _ _ _   _ _ _ _ _ _ _ _
    P E I A   O Y D A Z Q H A

    What tells you what time to start food preparation?

4. _ _ _ _ _
    P E I A N

    What should you set to help you remember how long food should be cooked?

5. _ _ _ _ _ _ _ _ _ _ _
    Z K R A P W E H E J C

    What is it called when you work on two tasks at the same time?

6. _ _ _   _ _ _ _ _
    D K P   S W P A N

    What should be used to rinse dishes?

7. _ _ _ _ _ _ _ _
    P A W I S K N G

    What is the key to success when working in the foods lab?

8. _ _ _ _ _ _ _ _ _ _ _ _ _ _
    N A O L K J O E X E H E P U

    What must each person in a group take?

9. _ _ _ _ _ _ _ _ _ _
    A R W H Q W P E K J

    What is the final step to take to complete lab work?

10. _ _ _ _   _ _ _ _ _ _ _ _ _ _   _ _ _ _ _
     C K K Z   I W J W C A I A J P   H A W Z O

     _ _   _ _ _ _ _ _ _   _ _   _ _ _
     P K   O Q Y Y A O O   E J   P D A

     _ _ _ _ _ _ _ .
     G E P Y D A J

CHAPTER 23

Text Pages 180-185

Conserving and Recycling

Study Guide

Directions: Answer the following questions on the lines provided.

1. What are two benefits of conserving fuel?

   _____

   _____

2. What happens to the amount of fuel used when an appliance is dirty or not working properly?

   _____

   _____

3. Why is a small appliance often more energy efficient for cooking than using the oven?

   _____

   _____

4. Why should you develop a habit of conserving water even when there is no shortage?

   _____

   _____

5. What are three suggestions for using less water?

   _____

   _____

   _____

6. How much trash does the average American create in a day?

   _____

7. Why should you look for products without much packaging?

   _____

   _____

Continued on next page

8. Give two suggestions to reduce the use of disposable products.

_____

_____

_____

9. Give three suggestions for reusing throwaway items.

_____

_____

_____

_____

10. Why is recycling a benefit to the community?

_____

_____

11. Describe how to prepare items for recycling.

_____

_____

_____

12. Why should you only buy as much food as you can use before it spoils?

_____

_____

CHAPTER 23
Conserving and Recycling

Be Conservation Conscious

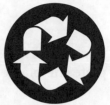

Directions: Read the story below about Jeremy and his mother. On the lines below, suggest ten ways that Jeremy and his mother could conserve or recycle resources.

"We're out of milk," called Jeremy to his mother as he tossed the plastic milk jug in the waste basket. She came into the kitchen and said, "I'll have to run to the supermarket before supper to get some. I just went to the store last night—I wish I'd gotten it then." As his mother got her keys and purse, Jeremy peeked in the oven and asked, "What's for dinner?" His mother said, "Meatloaf," as she went out the door. Jeremy held the oven door open for a minute, being warmed by the heat. He decided to get a drink of water. He turned on the water so it would cool and got a paper cup to drink from. As he filled the cup, he spilled some water on the floor. He got out a roll of pink plaid paper towels and wiped up the water. His mother walked in from the store. She had a jug of milk and a box of frozen corn for supper. After she took the groceries out of the bag, she handed the bag to Jeremy to throw away. "Will you set the table, Jeremy?" she said, "and I'll get the potatoes and corn heating on the cooktop."

1. _____

2. _____

3. _____

4. _____

5. _____

6. _____

7. _____

   _____

8. _____

   _____

9. _____

   _____

10. _____

    _____

Discovering Food and Nutrition Student Workbook

CHAPTER **23**

Conserving and Recycling

Conserve Our Resources

Directions: Listed below are clues that relate to conserving resources. Use each clue to complete the blank spaces in the corresponding numbered item.

1. ___ ___ ___ __ **C** __ __ __ __ __ __ __ __

2. ___ ___ ___ **O** __ __ __ __ __ __

3. ___ ___ ___ **N** __ __ __ __ __ __ __ __

4. ___ ___ ___ **S** __ __ __ __ __ __

5. ___ ___ ___ **E** __ __ __ __ __ __ __

6. ___ ___ **R** __ __ __ __ __ __ __ __

7. ___ **V** __ __ __

8. ___ **E** __ __ __ __ __ __

Clues

1. This makes up a large portion of trash.

2. This can create a water shortage.

3. A place where trash is normally buried.

4. This substance is made from petroleum.

5. This can pollute water if too much is used.

6. This will be improved by conserving and recycling.

7. Keep this door closed to save fuel when preparing food.

8. When people do this, new products are made from the materials of old ones.

CHAPTER 24
Meal Management

Study Guide

Directions: Answer the following questions on the lines provided.

1. Why are management skills useful in preparing meals?

   _____

   _____

2. What makes a good menu?

   _____

   _____

3. What are four points to keep in mind when planning menus and meals?

   _____

   _____

4. What are four ways you can bring variety to the foods in a menu?

   _____

   _____

5. What is lacking in this menu: Baked fish fillets; mashed potatoes; apple almond salad; milk?

   _____

   _____

6. How does the cook's choice of groceries affect meal preparation? Give an example.

   _____

   _____

   _____

7. Why is it important to identify preparation tasks when making a work plan?

   _____

   _____

Continued on next page

8. Would it be better to allow too much or too little time when estimating how much time is needed to complete each task in meal preparation? Why?

_____

_____

_____

_____

9. Why do most cooks work on several foods at once rather than preparing one, then another?

_____

_____

_____

10. Give examples of dovetailing tasks in meal preparation.

_____

_____

_____

11. How would you create a time schedule when planning your meal preparation?

_____

_____

_____

12. What is the purpose of evaluating your meal?

_____

_____

_____

CHAPTER 24

Meal Management

Cooking Consultant

Directions: Assume you write a newspaper column called *Cooking Consultant*. Read the following letters you have received and respond to the letters on the lines provided.

1. Dear CC:

My brother and I fix meals together, but we end up fighting. We try to help each other, but he'll have the utensil I need or I've already done what he is doing. Is there any way for us to work together?

Signed,
Kitchen Foes

_____

_____

_____

2. Dear CC:

I'm supposed to cook supper one night a week when my mom has to work late. I never manage to get everything ready at the same time—something is always burned, or cold, or only half cooked. How can I get things ready at the same time?

Signed,
Good Intentions

_____

_____

_____

3. Dear CC:

My favorite meal is chicken and noodles, applesauce, cauliflower, and French bread. Everyone groans when I fix it for supper. What's wrong with it?

Signed,
Puzzled

_____

_____

_____

CHAPTER **24**

Meal Management

Call for Successful Meal Planning

Directions: The numbers beneath the answer blanks below correspond to the numbers on the telephone buttons. There are three letters on each button (except the buttons marked 1 and 0). Decide which of the three letters on the indicated button is used in each answer. Write the correct letters in the spaces. If you decide on an answer from the clue alone, use the numbers to check your accuracy.

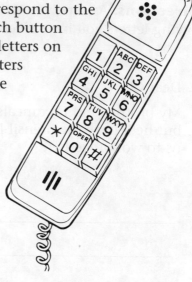

1. __ __ __ __ __ __ __ __
  7 5 2 6 6 4 6 4

Management skill used in preparing successful meals.

2. __ __ __ __
  6 3 6 8

A list of foods to serve at a meal.

3. __ __ __ __ __ __ __ __ __
  6 8 8 7 4 8 4 6 6

A very important factor to consider in planning meals.

4. __ __ __ __ __ __ __
  8 3 9 8 8 7 3

Whether a food is hard or soft.

5. __ __ __ __ __
  7 5 4 5 5

An example of a resource used in meal planning.

6. __ __ __ __ __ __ __
  3 5 2 8 6 7 7

A variety of these are desirable at each meal.

7. __ __ __ __ __
  2 6 5 6 7

Garnishes add this to a meal.

8. __ __ __ __ __ __ __ __
  9 6 7 5   7 5 2 6

Coordinating meal preparation is easier with this.

9. __ __ __ __ __ __ __ __ __ __ __ __
  6 3 2 5   7 2 8 8 3 7 6 7

People's preferences for eating certain foods at specific times of day.

CHAPTER 25 Seving a Meal

Study Guide

Directions: Answer the following questions on the lines provided.

1. What are the benefits of having a family routine at meal times?

   _____

   _____

2. What is the difference between family style and plate service?

   _____

   _____

   _____

3. When is buffet service often used?

   _____

   _____

4. What is tableware?

   _____

   _____

5. Why are tumblers generally used for family meals rather than stemware?

   _____

   _____

6. What is a place setting? What should be included in a place setting used with plate service?

   _____

   _____

   _____

7. Give an example of ordinary household items that can be used to decorate a table.

   _____

   _____

Continued on next page

8. How should flatware be placed when making a place setting?

_____

_____

_____

9. Why is it best to save disputes or problems until after mealtime?

_____

_____

10. What is the basis of good table manners?

_____

_____

11. When is it appropriate to start to eat when you are eating with a small group?

_____

_____

12. When and where should dishes be scraped and stacked?

_____

_____

Name _____ Date _____ Class Period _____

Using Tableware

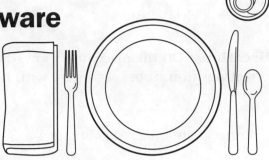

Directions: Read the menus listed below. On the lines provided, write the tableware you would use to serve the meal.

1. Grilled cheese sandwich, pasta salad, slice of watermelon, ice water, milk.

_____

_____

_____

_____

2. Lasagna, green tossed salad, garlic bread, chocolate pie, ice water, milk.

_____

_____

_____

_____

3. Potato soup, turkey sandwich, carrot and celery sticks, mixed fruit, hot cider.

_____

_____

_____

4. Pork chop, mashed potatoes, corn, gelatin salad, biscuits, ice water.

_____

_____

_____

5. Oatmeal, whole-wheat toast with peanut butter, orange juice, coffee.

_____

_____

_____

CHAPTER 25
Serving a Meal

Place Settings

Directions: On the placemat below, draw a place setting with each tableware item in the correct position. Label each item with its number.

1. dinner plate   2. salad plate   3. napkin   4. tumbler   5. cup and saucer

6. knife   7. dinner fork   8. salad fork   9. teaspoon

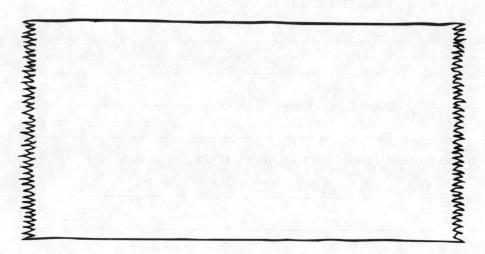

Directions: You are serving the menu listed below. Decide which tableware item or items your guests would use to eat each food. Write the numbers of the tableware needed next to each food item. Use the numbers from the place setting above.

Menu

_____ 10. Meatloaf

_____ 11. Twice-baked potato

_____ 12. Mixed vegetable casserole

_____ 13. Tossed salad

_____ 14. Wheat dinner rolls

_____ 15. Milk

CHAPTER 26

Packing a Lunch

Study Guide

Directions: Answer the following questions on the lines provided.

1. What can you do to be sure that you pack a nutritious lunch?

_____

_____

2. Why can sandwiches be a nutritious choice for a packed lunch?

_____

_____

3. Why is food safety a concern with packed lunches?

_____

_____

4. Why can using a vacuum bottle help keep food safe to eat?

_____

_____

5. What kind of lining in a vacuum bottle keeps hot foods the hottest?

_____

_____

6. Explain how to preheat a vacuum bottle.

_____

_____

_____

7. Why should a package of carrot and celery sticks be kept in the refrigerator until you are ready to pack your lunch?

_____

_____

Continued on next page

8. What are the advantages of making and freezing sandwiches ahead of time?

_____

_____

9. What do you need to do to keep your food fresh in a packed lunch?

_____

_____

10. How can you practice resource conservation when packing a lunch?

_____

_____

11. Explain how to prevent food odors in plastic containers.

_____

_____

12. Why should lettuce or tomato slices be packed separately and added to a sandwich just before eating it?

_____

_____

CHAPTER **26** Packing a Lunch

Lunch Online

Directions: Assume that you answer food-related questions on a website called Lunch Online. Read the e-mail you have received below and respond on the lines provided.

1. From Texas:

   I'm trying to eat more fruit and would like to take some apple juice or grape juice with my lunch. It doesn't taste good if it gets warm. How could I keep the juice cold?

   _____

   _____

2. From Indiana:

   I would rather take my lunch to school but I never seem to have time to pack it in the morning. I barely have time to grab some breakfast. How can I find time to make lunch?

   _____

   _____

3. From Georgia:

   I often carry fruit or salad in a plastic container. Lately I've noticed it has started to smell of food. Is there any way I can get rid of the smell?

   _____

   _____

4. From Colorado:

   I love sandwiches with mayonnaise, meat, lettuce, tomatoes, and other good vegetables on them. By lunchtime though the bread is so soggy I can't eat it. How can I prevent this from happening?

   _____

   _____

5. From Michigan:

   I often make a week's worth of sandwiches on the weekend and freeze them. This week I froze tuna and egg salad sandwiches. When I took them to school, they were awful! What did I do wrong?

   _____

   _____

CHAPTER 26

Packing a Lunch

Magic Lunch Square

Directions: Find the term that best fits each description. Write the number of the correct term in the space in each lettered square. If all your answers are correct, the total of the numbers, or the "Magic Number," will be the same in each row across and down. Write the Magic Number in the space provided.

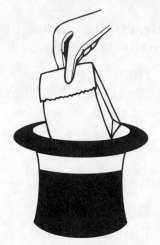

Terms

1. beverages

2. egg

3. heat source

4. illness

5. insulated bag

6. plastic container

7. preheated

8. safe

9. vacuum bottle

10. wide-mouthed

A	B	C
D	E	F
G	H	I

The Magic Number is _____.

Descriptions

A. What can occur if food in a packed lunch is not kept either cold or very hot.

B. This sandwich filling does not freeze well.

C. A container used to keep foods at their original temperature.

D. Avoid storing a packed lunch near this.

E. What should be done to a vacuum bottle before carrying soup in it.

F. This can be used to keep a packed lunch cold.

G. A packed lunch needs to be this.

H. This helps keep packed food fresh.

I. What is usually carried in a narrow-mouth vacuum bottle.

CHAPTER 27 Milk

Study Guide

Directions: Answer the following questions on the lines provided.

1. Why is milk one of the most nutritious beverages you can drink? How many servings from this food group should you have each day?

   _____

   _____

2. What kind of milk is recommended for children younger than age two? Why?

   _____

   _____

3. How does a consumer decide which form of milk to buy?

   _____

   _____

4. Why should all milk you drink be pasteurized?

   _____

   _____

5. Does fat-free milk need to be homogenized? Explain your answer.

   _____

   _____

   _____

6. What vitamins are frequently added to fat-free milk? What benefits do they bring the consumer?

   _____

   _____

7. What does the date on the package of milk mean?

   _____

   _____

Continued on next page

8. How is evaporated milk used?

_____

_____

9. Why should a skin that forms over heated milk be stirred back into the milk?

_____

_____

10. List three ways you might use a white sauce when cooking.

_____

_____

_____

11. What is one advantage of heating milk in the microwave?

_____

_____

12. Why would you add nonfat dry milk to recipes that don't call for it?

_____

_____

CHAPTER 27 Milk

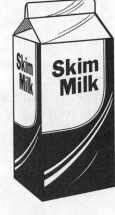

Milk Choices

Directions: Read each situation described below. Answer the question on the lines provided.

1. Dane is heating tomato soup. When he checked the soup, it had separated into many small lumps and a watery liquid. What happened to the milk in the soup? Why?

_____

_____

2. A recipe that Shawonda wants to make calls for sweetened condensed milk. She has a can of evaporated milk. Can she make this substitution and have a successful product? Why or why not?

_____

_____

_____

3. Devon has made pudding that has a burnt flavor. What may have caused this? How could she have prevented it?

_____

_____

_____

4. A recipe Gabe is using says to reconstitute nonfat dry milk. What does this mean?

_____

_____

5. Allison is considering buying whole milk. Is this a good choice if she is trying to gain weight? Why?

_____

_____

Cooking with Milk

Directions: What is the nutrient in milk that makes it sensitive to heat? To discover the answer, write the word or phrase for each definition or question in the blanks provided, placing one letter on each blank. Transfer the circled letter to the appropriate blank in #8 below.

1. _ _ _ _O_ _   Stir white sauce constantly to prevent these.

2. _ _ _ _ _ _ _ _O_   What milk does if not stirred when heated in the microwave.

3. _ _O_ _ _ _   Can be made from a thin cream sauce.

4. _ _ _O_ _   A milk-based sauce thickened with flour.

5. _ _O_ _ _ _   The kind of texture a cooked milk product should have.

6. _ _O_ _   This kind of ingredient can cause milk to curdle.

7. _ _ _ _O   What milk solids do if cooked at too high a temperature.

8. _ _ _ _ _ _ _ _

Directions: Milk will have a burnt flavor if not cooked correctly. What is the first step in preventing this? To discover the answer, write the word or phrase for each definition or question on the blanks to its left, placing one letter on each blank. Transfer the circled letters to the appropriate blanks in #19 below.

9. _ _O_ _ _   Milk is often used in recipes for these.

10. O_ _ _ _ _   How milk should be cooked.

11. _ _O_ _   This is prevented from escaping by a milk skin.

12. _ _ _ _O_   What milk does when it separates into tiny lumps and a watery liquid.

13. _O_ _ _ _ _ _ _   Milk is likely to do this when heated in the microwave. (2 words)

14. _ _ _O_   What milk skin usually is.

15. _ _ _ _ _O_ _   Milk that has a burnt flavor.

16. _ _O_ _   This may help prevent a milk skin from forming.

17. _ _ _ _ _O_   Milk is less likely to scorch in this.

18. _ _O_   This is part of what makes up a milk skin.

19. _ _ _ _ _ _ _ _ _ _ _

CHAPTER 28
Yogurt and Cheese

Study Guide

Directions: Answer the following questions on the lines provided.

1. What gives yogurt its texture and flavor?

   _____

   _____

2. What are the basic steps in making cheese?

   _____

   _____

3. Why are yogurt and cheese good menu choices for people who cannot or don't like to drink milk?

   _____

   _____

4. What nutrient is more likely to be found in cheese than in yogurt?

   _____

   _____

5. What is the difference between yogurt and frozen yogurt?

   _____

   _____

6. What is a major difference between ripened and unripened cheese?

   _____

   _____

7. How are process and cold-pack cheeses made?

   _____

   _____

Continued on next page

8. You are looking at two different brands of mozzarella cheese in the store. They are in the same sized packages and cost the same. How might you decide between them?

_____

_____

9. What is the benefit of substituting low-fat yogurt cheese for cream cheese?

_____

_____

10. What should you do to ripened cheese before eating to improve its taste?

_____

_____

11. How long should cheese generally be cooked? Why?

_____

_____

12. What happens to cheese that is overcooked in the microwave?

_____

_____

Name _____ Date _____ Class Period _____

CHAPTER 28 Yogurt and Cheese

Cheese Clues

Directions: Hidden in this puzzle are the nine kinds of cheese listed in scrambled form below. Unscramble the letters and then circle the cheese names in the puzzle. Names will appear backward, forward, horizontally, and vertically. Then list each cheese in the appropriate column below.

daehdcr _____   necmiraa _____

dareps _____   sissw _____

krcbi _____   tgetoca _____

marce _____   tgyuor _____

meanraps _____

```
S   O   P   A   R   M   E   S   A   N
W   A   W   M   E   S   M   I   C   R
I   C   H   E   D   D   A   R   R   E
S   P   A   R   A   T   E   R   E   A
S   S   O   I   S   P   R   E   A   D
B   R   I   C   K   O   C   R   M   A
T   E   G   A   T   T   O   C   R   S
S   W   I   N   T   R   U   G   O   Y
```

1. Unripened   **2. Ripened**   **3. Process**

_____   _____   _____

_____   _____   _____

_____   _____   _____

_____   _____   _____

CHAPTER 28
Yogurt and Cheese

Choosing Cheese and Yogurt

Directions: Read the situations below, make any necessary calculations, and answer the questions in the space provided.

1. Your friend wants to consume more calcium and has decided to try yogurt. She changed her mind because the label of the yogurt she considered buying said that it contained "live cultures." What would you tell her?

_____

_____

_____

2. You are planning to make a casserole in the microwave tonight. You would like to top it with a little cheese. In the refrigerator, you have process American cheese slices, cream cheese, shredded cheddar, and a carton of cottage cheese. Which would you use? How would you cook it?

_____

_____

_____

_____

3. Erin plans to serve cheese slices and fruit to her friends while they work on a school project. At the supermarket she can't decide what cheese to buy. She is considering individually wrapped American cheese slices that cost $3.49 for a 16 oz. package. She also sees a variety package of sliced cheddar, brick, and Swiss cheese that costs $2.65 for 8 oz.; a 10 oz. block of sharp cheddar that costs $2.75; and an 8 oz. package of sliced cheddar that costs $2.49. What is the cost per ounce of each option? What would you buy? Why?

_____

_____

_____

_____

CHAPTER 29   Grain Products

Study Guide

Directions: Answer the following questions on the lines provided.

1. Why are foods in the Bread, Cereal, Rice, and Pasta group so important in the diet? List three food products that are made from grains.

   _____

   _____

   _____

   _____

2. What kind of protein is found in grain products? What does this mean in terms of your diet?

   _____

   _____

3. What are the three main parts of a grain kernel? What nutrients are found in each part?

   _____

   _____

   _____

4. Why are whole grain products more nutritious than products made from only the endosperm?

   _____

   _____

   _____

5. What is the best way to add fiber to your diet?

   _____

   _____

6. Why is it important to look at the nutrition labels when buying breakfast cereals?

   _____

   _____

Continued on next page

7. How does brown rice differ from enriched rice?

_____

_____

_____

_____

8. How is pasta made?

_____

_____

9. Is it better to store bread at room temperature or in the refrigerator? Why?

_____

_____

10. Describe a properly cooked grain product.

_____

_____

11. Should you rinse grain products after cooking? Why or why not?

_____

_____

12. How does the cooking time for grains vary when cooked on the rangetop and cooked in the microwave?

_____

_____

Text Pages 222-231

CHAPTER 29

Grain Products

Grains and Breads Puzzle

Directions: Listed below are clues that have to do with grains, breads, and a healthful diet. Fill in the letter blanks for each term to complete the puzzle.

1. __ __ __ G __ __ __ __ __ __

2. __ __ R __ __ __ __

3. __ __ __ A

4. __ I B __ __

5. __ N R __ __ __ __ __

6. __ S E __ __

7. __ A __ __ __

8. __ __ __ __ __ D

9. __ __ __ __ S __ __ __

Clues

1. You increase fat and calories when you serve bread with this.

2. A thin, flat bread made from corn flour or wheat flour.

3. A thick, flat bread with a pocket.

4. Whole-grain breads are a good source of this.

5. Bread that has added iron and B vitamins.

6. Another name for the kernels of cereal grains.

7. A donut-shaped roll with a chewy texture.

8. The way most loaves of bread are sold.

9. All-purpose white flour is made from this.

CHAPTER 29   Grain Products

How Much Is Too Much?

Directions: Grain products increase in bulk when they are cooked. Pasta generally swells to double in size while rice triples in size. In answering the following questions, assume that one serving equals 1/2 cup.

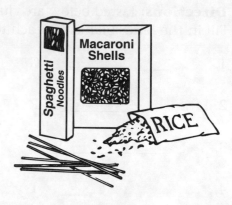

1. Stephanie's recipe for pasta salad calls for 4 cups of cooked rotini. She places 4 cups of uncooked rotini in boiling water. How much rotini will she end up with? What will she have to do to the recipe if she uses all of the pasta?

_____

2. A recipe for a chicken casserole calls for 3 cups of cooked noodles. How many cups of uncooked noodles would you need to use?

_____

3. How much uncooked macaroni would be needed to serve ten people?

_____

4. How much uncooked spaghetti would be needed to serve four people?

_____

5. A recipe for a beef casserole calls for 3 cups of cooked rice. How much raw rice would you cook?

_____

6. How much uncooked rice would be needed to serve 12 people?

_____

7. How much uncooked rice would be needed to serve two people?

_____

CHAPTER 30 Fruits

Study Guide

Directions: Answer the following questions on the lines provided.

1. How many servings of fruit should you eat each day?

   _____

   _____

2. Why are fruits an important part of a healthful diet?

   _____

   _____

   _____

3. Why can the price of fresh fruit vary dramatically over time?

   _____

   _____

4. Why is it important to know whether a fruit continues to ripen after it is picked?

   _____

   _____

   _____

5. Explain the statement from the text: "Low quality fruits are no bargain."

   _____

   _____

   _____

Continued on next page

6. Describe the characteristics of a high-quality grapefruit.

_____

_____

_____

7. You have bought fresh blueberries. How would you store them when you got home?

_____

_____

_____

8. Why does a recipe for banana pudding tell you to put a tablespoon of lemon juice on the sliced bananas before adding them to the pudding?

_____

_____

9. If you wanted to serve frozen strawberries on angel food cake for dessert, would you thaw the strawberries completely before putting them on the cake? Why or why not?

_____

_____

10. If you wanted cooked sliced apples to hold their shape, when should you add the sugar to them? Why?

_____

_____

11. Why do fruits cook quickly in the microwave? Why is this an advantage?

_____

_____

12. What can you do to prevent a fruit from bursting in the microwave? Why does this work?

_____

_____

_____

Name _____ Date _____ Class Period _____

Choosing Nutritious Fruits

Directions: It is important to consider nutrition when choosing fruit. Listed below are pairs of fruits. Put a check in the blank to the left of the fruit in each pair you think is the best choice. Explain why in the space provided.

1. _____ Frozen strawberries with sugar

   _____ Frozen strawberries without sugar

   Explain your choice.

   _____

   _____

   _____

2. _____ Fresh grapefruit segments

   _____ Canned grapefruit segments

   Explain your choice.

   _____

   _____

   _____

3. _____ Fresh apple

   _____ Freshly-made applesauce

   Explain your choice.

   _____

   _____

   _____

CHAPTER 30   Fruits

Consumer Power

Directions: Read each question below. Make any calculations on a separate sheet of paper and answer the questions on the lines provided.

1. Packaged apples come in a tray of four for $1.59. What is the cost per apple?

   _____

2. Loose apples are on sale at three for $1.00. What is the cost per apple?

   _____

3. Which is the better buy, loose or packaged apples?

   _____

   _____

4. A 15-ounce jar of applesauce costs $1.05. What is the cost per ounce?

   _____

5. A 48-ounce jar of applesauce costs $2.39. What is the cost per ounce?

   _____

6. Which jar of applesauce is the better buy?

   _____

   _____

7. A 15-ounce box of raisins costs $1.54. What is the cost per ounce?

   _____

8. A pack of six 1-ounce boxes costs $1.15. What is the cost per ounce?

   _____

9. Which has a lower unit cost, the large box of raisins or the six small packages?

   _____

10. Sometimes the best buy is not the best choice for you. Other than price, what factors might you think about in buying fruit?

    _____

    _____

CHAPTER 31
Vegetables

Study Guide

Directions: Answer the following questions on the lines provided.

1. Why are vegetables a healthful part of daily food choices? How many servings of vegetables are recommended each day?

_____

_____

_____

2. What vitamins and minerals can be found in vegetables?

_____

_____

3. From what parts of the plant do the following vegetables come: celery, corn, eggplant, and beets?

_____

_____

4. What form of vegetables generally contains the most nutrients?

_____

_____

5. What is the advantage of buying locally grown vegetables when they are in season?

_____

_____

6. You are looking at green peppers in the supermarket. Most of them are a pale green. They seem soft and appear somewhat wilted. Would you buy one? Why or why not?

_____

_____

_____

Continued on next page

7. Identify four ways vegetables can be included in daily menus.

_____

_____

8. Why should the outer parts of vegetables not be pared away unless they are damaged?

_____

_____

9. Describe vegetables that have been overcooked.

_____

_____

10. Why is making a stir-fry a good way to include vegetables in your diet?

_____

_____

11. How much water should be used when simmering vegetables? Why is this amount recommended?

_____

_____

12. Why is microwaving a healthful method for cooking vegetables?

_____

_____

CHAPTER 31 Vegetables

Vegetables and Nutrients

Directions: Read the situations described below.
Answer each question on the lines provided.

1. James is on a low-calorie diet. Why are vegetables a good food choice for him?

_____

_____

_____

2. Kayla is allergic to milk. What vegetables could she eat to help her get enough calcium in her diet?

_____

_____

3. Brett doesn't care for oranges and grapefruit. His mother encourages him to get more vitamin C. What vegetables could he eat that contain vitamin C?

_____

_____

_____

4. Sierra wants to get the most nutrients possible in the vegetables she buys. Should she buy fresh, frozen, or canned?

_____

_____

_____

5. Miranda usually microwaves vegetables. She wonders if this is a good way to save nutrients? Is it? Why or why not?

_____

_____

CHAPTER **31**

Vegetables

Steps to a Perfect Vegetable Tray

Directions: Tony is buying fresh vegetables to make a vegetable tray for a party. Follow Tony's steps from the supermarket and at home. Answer the questions about how Tony should choose, store, and prepare the vegetables on the lines below.

1. What qualities should Tony look for in choosing the vegetables?

_____

_____

_____

2. When Tony gets home, how should he store the vegetables?

_____

_____

_____

3. On the day of the party, how should Tony prepare the vegetables for the tray?

_____

_____

_____

4. How should Tony store the prepared vegetables to keep them crisp until it is time for the party?

_____

_____

_____

CHAPTER 32

Legumes

Study Guide

Directions: Answer the following questions on the lines provided.

1. What are legumes? Give two examples of legumes.

_____

_____

_____

_____

2. What minerals can be found in legumes?

_____

_____

3. What beans are typically used in Mexican foods? Middle Eastern foods?

_____

_____

4. Why is tofu considered a healthful food?

_____

_____

5. How long does tofu need to be cooked?

_____

_____

6. How can cooked legumes be stored for several weeks?

_____

_____

7. How can you reduce the amount of sodium found in canned beans?

_____

_____

Continued on next page

8. What are the three steps in preparing dry beans?

_____

_____

9. What are the benefits of soaking beans overnight before cooking?

_____

_____

10. How long are beans normally simmered?

_____

_____

11. What will happen if you add salt or sugar to the water when preparing to cook beans?

_____

_____

12. Will a microwave shorten cooking time when preparing dried beans? Explain your answer.

_____

_____

CHAPTER 32
Legumes

Solving Legume Problems

Directions: Read each situation described below. Answer the questions on the lines provided.

1. Adam cooked dried pinto beans for supper. He cooked them like he cooks green beans—for 10 minutes in the microwave. No one could eat the pinto beans. What did Adam do wrong?

   _____

   _____

2. Lateesha is making dinner for her family. Her mother told her to use the rest of the tofu in the refrigerator. She had planned to serve a Mexican casserole made with ground beef, tortilla chips and dip, and a green salad. How might Lateesha use up the tofu with this menu?

   _____

   _____

   _____

3. Connor has been put on a low-sodium diet for his blood pressure. He has always eaten a lot of canned beans. Can he continue to eat them on his diet? Explain your answer.

   _____

   _____

4. Danielle is cooking dried black-eyed peas for supper. She uses the last of an opened package and opens a new package to have enough for her family. When she eats her serving, she discovers that some of the peas are tender while some are not. What could have caused this problem?

   _____

   _____

5. The soup recipe Jesse made called for ½ cup cooked kidney beans. He decided to just cook the beans in the soup, so he put the ½ cup of dried beans directly in the broth. When the soup was done, there were way too many beans in it. Why did this happen?

   _____

   _____

   _____

CHAPTER 32	Text Pages 248-255

Legumes

Legume Calculations

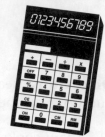

Directions: Fill in the chart by calculating price per ounce of the legumes listed below. Then answer the questions on the lines provided.

Legume	Processing	Size	Cost	Unit Cost
Great Northern Beans	Dried	2 lb.	$0.86	1. _____
Great Northern Beans	Canned	15 oz.	$0.51	2. _____
Kidney Beans	Dried	1 lb.	$0.68	3. _____
Kidney Beans	Canned	15 oz.	$0.56	4. _____

5. Is it accurate to directly compare unit prices of dried and canned beans? Explain.

_____

_____

_____

_____

6. The canned beans are about the same price. How would you decide which to buy?

_____

_____

7. What are the advantages of buying dried legumes?

_____

_____

_____

8. What are the advantages of buying canned legumes?

_____

_____

CHAPTER 33 Poultry

Study Guide

Directions: Answer the following questions on the lines provided.

1. Why is poultry a popular main-dish food?

_____

_____

2. Where is most of the fat located in chicken and turkey? How can you avoid eating it?

_____

_____

3. What are two ways of preparing poultry that add no fat during the cooking process?

_____

_____

4. How does the dark meat differ from white meat in a turkey?

_____

_____

5. What kinds of cooking methods would be appropriate for a chicken labeled a "broiler."

_____

_____

6. How can you use the cost per serving formula when buying poultry?

_____

_____

7. Where should poultry be stored in the refrigerator?

_____

_____

8. What does it mean if the label on a package of turkey bacon says it is cured?

_____

_____

Continued on next page

9. Why is food safety so important when working with raw poultry?

_____

_____

10. How should you thaw frozen poultry?

_____

_____

11 Why should you use a meat thermometer when cooking poultry?

_____

_____

_____

12. Why is braising a good method for cooking stewing chickens?

_____

_____

13. Why does fried chicken usually have more calories than broiled chicken?

_____

_____

14. How should chicken be arranged when you are cooking it in the microwave oven?

_____

_____

CHAPTER 33 Poultry

Shopping for Poultry

Directions: Read the situations described below. Answer each question on the lines provided.

1. Mark wanted to fry chicken for supper. Hens were on sale at the supermarket, so he bought one. What word would most likely describe the fried hen he made?

_____

_____

_____

2. Jasmine is looking at chicken breasts. The boneless chicken breasts are $3.99 a pound. The split chicken breasts contain the chicken breast bone but cost $2.49 a pound. Which is the better buy to serve four people? Why?

_____

_____

_____

3. Madison is looking at two whole chickens. One is labeled Grade A and one is Grade B. What is the difference between the two grades?

_____

_____

4. Justin often buys ground turkey instead of ground beef because he believes it is lower in fat. He has learned that the meat market where he shops puts turkey skin in the ground turkey. What affect does this have on the fat content of the ground turkey?

_____

_____

5. Hayley always buys pieces of chicken with the bones in them because they are so much less expensive than the boneless. Is she actually saving money?

_____

_____

_____

Name _____ Date _____ Class Period _____

Poultry Math

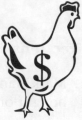

Directions: Read the situations below and write your calculations in the box under each situation. Write your answers on the lines provided on the right-hand side of each box.

1. Beth is buying 3 pounds of chicken thighs for $1.29 per pound. How much will she pay? How many servings will the thighs provide?

```



                                                            _____
```

2. Dan is buying turkey cutlets for $2.69 per pound. The package weighs 4 pounds, 8 ounces. How much will the cutlets cost?

```



                                                            _____
```

3. Kyle bought a 2 pound (1000 g) fryer for $1.19 a pound. How many servings will the fryer make? What will his cost per serving be?

```



                                                            _____
```

4. Michael is having 12 people at his house for a family dinner. He wants to roast a turkey. How large a turkey would he need to serve everyone? He'd also like to buy 4 pounds extra for turkey sandwiches. If turkey costs $1.19 per pound, how much would a turkey big enough for dinner and sandwiches cost?

```



                                                            _____
```

CHAPTER 34
Fish and Shellfish

Study Guide

Directions: Answer the following questions on the lines provided.

1. What is the difference between fish and shellfish?

   _____

   _____

   _____

2. Why are fish a healthful addition to the diet?

   _____

   _____

   _____

3. If you wanted boneless fish, would you buy steaks or fillets? Why?

   _____

   _____

   _____

4. What is the advantage of buying shucked shellfish?

   _____

   _____

5. What is surimi? How is it made?

   _____

   _____

   _____

6. What qualities should you look for when buying fresh fish?

   _____

   _____

Continued on next page

7. What should you look for when buying frozen fish?

_____

_____

8. If shrimp in the shell is $9.99 a pound, how much would a serving cost?

_____

9. Why should fish be cooked thoroughly before eating?

_____

_____

10. You decide to cook fish fillets while they are still frozen. How do you adjust the recipe?

_____

_____

11. Why is fish a naturally tender food?

_____

_____

12. When broiling fish, how far away from the heat source should the pan be? Why should thin fish fillets not be broiled?

_____

_____

13. What is the 10-minute rule for cooking fish?

_____

_____

14. What is the advantage of a crumb coating on fish when cooking the fish in the microwave?

_____

_____

15. Why should fish stand for 5 to 10 minutes after being cooked in a microwave oven?

_____

_____

CHAPTER 34   Fish and Shellfish

Fishy Calculations

Directions: Read the problems below and calculate the answers to each question. In the blank to the left of the question, write the letter of the fish that contains the answer to the problem.

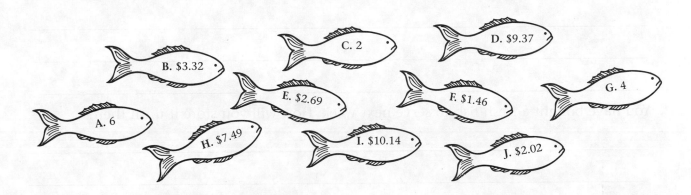

_____ 1. Jason bought cod fillets for dinner. The cod cost $4.99 per pound and had a net weight of 1 lb. 8 oz. How much did Jason pay for the fish?

_____ 2. The fresh red snapper fillets Lauren was looking at cost $4.39 per pound. If she bought 3 pounds, how much would the fillets cost per serving?

_____ 3. Andy needs 24 oz. of tuna for a casserole. The 6 oz. cans cost $0.83 and the 12 oz. cans cost $2.09. What would he pay if he buys the most economical size?

_____ 4. Michelle caught a 4 lb. trout on a fishing trip. How many servings will the fish provide?

_____ 5. Tim bought 2 pounds of pollock at $2.99 per pound and a can of red salmon for $3.39. How much was his total bill?

_____ 6. Luis bought 2 pounds of salmon steaks at $6.99 per pound. How many servings will the steaks make?

_____ 7. Alyssa bought a package of frozen perch for $3.49, and 1 lb. of orange roughy for $4.49. She gave the grocery clerk $10.00. How much change did she get back?

CHAPTER 34

Fish and Shellfish

What Would You Do?

Directions: Read each situation described below. Answer the questions on the lines provided.

1. You've decided to try to increase your intake of calcium. What fish could you eat to accomplish this goal?

_____

_____

_____

2. You have bought a fresh fish to serve next week. How will you store it until then?

_____

_____

3. You like shellfish, but have never prepared it before. Your store has fresh crab and crab-flavored surimi. If they cost about the same per pound, which would you buy? Why?

_____

_____

_____

_____

4. The fish you prepared is dry and mealy. It fell apart when you tried to eat it with your fork. What would you do next time to avoid this problem?

_____

_____

5. You want to try broiling fish for the first time. What steps would you take to do this?

_____

_____

_____

_____

CHAPTER 35 Meat

Study Guide

Directions: Answer the following questions on the lines provided.

1. What are the main nutrients in meat?

_____

_____

2. Why is the recommended amount of meat often limited in low-fat diets?

_____

_____

3. How much does a serving of meat weigh?

_____

_____

4. What is the difference between beef and veal?

_____

_____

5. What is a cut of meat? What type of cuts do consumers buy?

_____

_____

6. Why is it important to know the cut of a piece of meat before you cook it?

_____

_____

7. What kind of tissue can make meat tough?

_____

_____

8. Explain what marbling is.

_____

_____

Continued on next page

9. Which grade of meat is the most expensive? What makes it more expensive?

_____

_____

10. What affects the number of servings you can get from a cut of meat?

_____

_____

11. Why are cuts of meat with a large amount of bone and fat often not economical even though they may have a low price per pound?

_____

_____

12. Give two examples of cured meats.

_____

_____

13. How do you check to see if a hamburger is thoroughly cooked? What internal temperature indicates that meat has been cooked enough to be safe to eat?

_____

_____

14. Why should the fat on the edges of a piece of meat be slashed before broiling?

_____

_____

15. What kinds of cuts of meat cook best in the microwave?

_____

_____

CHAPTER 35 Meat

How Much Does a Serving Cost?

Directions: Listed below are several cuts of meat and their cost per pound. Also given are the number of servings the meat provides per pound. Figure the cost per serving for each meat and answer the question below on the lines provided.

Cut of Meat	Cost Per Pound	Servings per Pound	Cost per Serving
Beef			
Ground Beef (lean)	$2.19	4	1. _____
Ground Beef (regular)	$1.79	4	2. _____
Sirloin Steak	$4.19	4	3. _____
Bottom Round Roast	$2.59	3	4. _____
Lamb			
Loin Chop	$6.29	3	5. _____
Shoulder Roast	$2.99	3	6. _____
Leg of Lamb Steak	$3.79	3	7. _____
Pork			
Bacon	$2.99	4	8. _____
Ham (boneless)	$4.29	4	9. _____
Loin Chop	$2.49	3	10. _____

11. What was the most expensive meat per pound? _____

12. Why do you think this cut was most expensive? _____

_____

13. What was the least expensive meat per pound? _____

14. Why do you think this cut was least expensive? _____

_____

_____

15. What conclusions can you draw from this activity? _____

_____

_____

_____

Discovering Food and Nutrition Student Workbook

| **CHAPTER 35** Meat | **Text Pages 278-291** |

LOOK at the Label

Directions: Shown below is a label from a package of meat. Read the label and answer the questions on the lines provided.

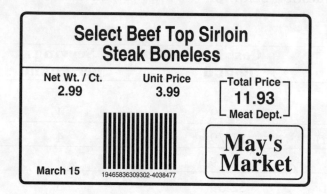

1. What kind of meat is in this package?_____

2. How much does this meat cost per pound? _____

3. How much does the meat in this package weigh? _____

4. What is the price of this package of meat?_____

5. What does the date on the label mean? _____

   _____

6. What is the retail cut of this meat?_____

7. What grade is this meat? _____

8. Is this a tender or a less-tender cut of meat? _____

9. What are two ways you could cook this piece of meat?

   _____

   _____

10. How many servings could you get from this package of meat? _____

    _____

Study Guide

Directions: Answer the following questions on the lines provided.

1. Why do health experts recommend eating no more than four eggs a week?

   _____

   _____

2. Why should you avoid any food products that may have been made with raw eggs?

   _____

   _____

3. What are the three purposes eggs can serve in recipes?

   _____

   _____

4. Why should you always break an egg into a small bowl?

   _____

   _____

5. Can egg whites that contain a small amount of egg yolk be beaten satisfactorily? Explain your answer.

   _____

   _____

6. Why should beaten egg whites be handled gently?

   _____

   _____

7. In what types of foods is a meringue generally used?

   _____

   _____

Continued on next page

8. At what temperature should eggs be cooked? Why?

_____

_____

9. What are the advantages and disadvantages of frying eggs?

_____

_____

_____

10. How are poached eggs cooked?

_____

_____

11. Why should you not cook eggs in the shell in the microwave? What should you do to a whole egg yolk before microwaving? Why?

_____

_____

_____

12. Which part of the egg cooks fastest in the microwave? Explain how to successfully cook an egg in the microwave.

_____

_____

CHAPTER 36 Eggs

Buying Eggs

Directions: Answer the following
questions on the lines provided.

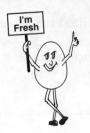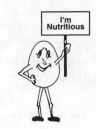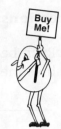

1. Curt is buying eggs for baking a cake
   and some cookies. Large eggs cost 92
   cents a dozen while small eggs are 79
   cents a dozen. Which size eggs should
   he buy? Why?

   _____

   _____

2. Carrie is looking at eggs in the supermarket. The store is having a sale on eggs and has
   extra cartons of eggs sitting in the aisle beside the refrigerated egg case. Does it matter if
   Carrie takes her carton from the aisle display or the refrigerator case? Why?

   _____

   _____

3. Emma is buying eggs for her family's use. The large eggs cost 99 cents a dozen while the
   medium eggs cost 90 cents. Which eggs are of better quality? Why?

   _____

   _____

4. It usually takes Brad about a month to use a carton of eggs. He's thinking about buying
   three cartons while they are on sale. Should Brad do this? Why or why not?

   _____

   _____

5. The supermarket where Tracy is shopping has cracked eggs for 1/2 price. Should she buy
   them? Why?

   _____

   _____

CHAPTER **36** Eggs

Using and Cooking Eggs

Directions: Read each situation described below. Answer the questions on the lines provided.

1. Ryan became very ill after eating homemade ice cream. Could the ice cream have caused his illness? Explain your answer.

   _____

   _____

2. Kiara is making a salmon loaf. The recipe calls for an egg. Kiara thinks it is odd that a salmon loaf would contain an egg. Why is the egg included in the recipe?

   _____

   _____

3. Cody cracked an egg on the side of a bowl in which he was mixing cookies. He got eggshell in the cookie batter when he added the egg. What should he have done to prevent this?

   _____

   _____

   _____

4. Katherine is making a meringue for a pie. The recipe says to beat until the egg whites form soft peaks. What should Katherine use to beat the eggs? How will they look when they reach the soft peak stage?

   _____

   _____

   _____

5. Alec wanted to make scrambled eggs. He put the eggs in the pan and stirred them. Then he let them cook. He was very disappointed with the results because the eggs looked like a flat pancake. What should he have done? Why?

   _____

   _____

CHAPTER 37 Salads

Study Guide

Directions: Answer the following questions on the lines provided.

1. What ingredients could you add to a salad to provide vitamins and minerals?

   _____

   _____

   _____

2. In making a salad, what ingredients could you add that would provide fiber and complex carbohydrates?

   _____

   _____

   _____

3. What would be good sources of protein to add to greens to make a main dish salad?

   _____

   _____

   _____

4. Why should small amounts of egg and cheese be used in salads?

   _____

   _____

5. What should you look for when choosing a salad dressing?

   _____

   _____

6. Why would you use a variety of greens rather than just one kind when making a salad?

   _____

   _____

Continued on next page

7. What are the three parts of most salads?

_____

_____

8. Explain how to core iceberg lettuce.

_____

_____

_____

9. What two purposes do dressings serve when making a salad? When should dressing be added to a green salad? Why?

_____

_____

_____

10. Why should the ingredients be dry before making a salad?

_____

_____

11. Why is it better to tear greens into bite-size pieces than to cut them?

_____

_____

12. What makes a molded salad different from other types of salads? From what ingredient is a molded salad usually made?

_____

_____

DISCOVERING FOOD AND NUTRITION Student Workbook

Name _____ Date _____ Class Period _____

A Tossed Salad

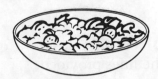

Directions: Fifteen ingredients for a salad have been "tossed" into the hidden word puzzle below. The ingredients are printed forward, backward, horizontally, and vertically. Circle each ingredient and list it under the appropriate heading below.

```
A  S  D  E  E  S  R  E  W  O  L  F  N  U  S  M  G  I
Y  N  L  R  E  X  O  N  I  F  T  Q  U  H  R  P  R  C
S  I  D  S  C  J  M  C  A  R  R  O  T  S  E  N  E  K
P  S  J  L  U  Y  A  R  A  G  E  N  I  V  B  R  E  H
I  I  W  C  T  T  I  W  E  A  V  K  M  R  M  O  N  E
N  A  B  H  T  O  N  Q  I  T  B  N  G  A  U  W  P  S
A  R  I  C  E  B  E  R  G  L  E  T  T  U  C  E  E  C
C  L  U  V  L  O  N  I  O  N  S  H  C  G  U  R  P  A
H  O  W  M  F  D  E  S  N  O  T  U  O  R  C  A  P  R
N  O  N  F  A  T  Y  O  G  U  R  T  T  M  A  I  E  O
Y  A  L  N  E  C  I  U  J  N  O  M  E  L  T  K  R  L
K  C  S  A  L  F  O  T  F  A  S  T  E  O  U  T  S  E
```

Greens	Vegetables	Toppings	Dressing
_____	_____	_____	_____
_____	_____	_____	_____
_____	_____	_____	_____
_____	_____		
_____			

CHAPTER 37 Salads

Making a Salad

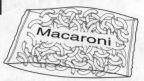

Directions: Read the questions below. Answer each on the lines provided.

1. Imagine that you want to make a main dish salad for lunch. You have found a recipe that calls for leaf lettuce, diced ham, pineapple chunks, tomato chunks, slices of carrot, and a low-fat sweet and sour dressing. What nutrients would be contained in the salad?

   _____

   _____

2. How would you store the leaf lettuce when you get the heads home from the store?

   _____

   _____

3. What is the purpose of the salad dressing in the recipe?

   _____

   _____

4. What should you look for on the salad dressing label when you are buying the low-fat sweet and sour dressing?

   _____

   _____

5. Identify the following parts of the salad you are making: base, body, dressing.

   _____

   _____

   _____

6. If you want to eat lunch at noon, when should you prepare the salad? Why?

   _____

   _____

Text Pages 310-315

CHAPTER 38 Soups

Study Guide

Directions: Answer the following questions on the lines provided.

1. What is meant by a hearty soup?

   _____

   _____

2. What ingredients are usually included in chowder?

   _____

   _____

3. Why is the broth in soup a good source of nutrients?

   _____

   _____

4. What ingredient could you add to soup that would provide both fiber and protein?

   _____

5. How can you make sure a soup is low in fat?

   _____

   _____

6. What are the benefits of using canned and frozen soups?

   _____

   _____

   _____

7. What is bouillon?

   _____

   _____

Continued on next page

8. What are two ways you can use good management when making soup?

_____

_____

_____

9. What is the advantage of adding your own ingredients to convenience soups?

_____

_____

10. What is the base for most cream soups?

_____

_____

11. List two herbs or spices that could be used to season homemade soup.

_____

_____

12. Why should soups be stirred once or twice while being heated in the microwave?

_____

_____

CHAPTER **38**

Soups

Soup with Sam

Directions: Assume you are a food columnist named Sam. The topic for your column today is Soup Savvy. You have received the letters below. Answer the letters on the lines provided.

1. Dear Sam,

Help! I tried my best to make a good chicken broth, but it's full of fat. No one will want to eat it like this. Is there anything I can do besides throw it out?

_____

_____

_____

2. Dear Sam,

I made some creamy vegetable soup with a white sauce and carrots, celery, and potatoes. The soup curdled long before the vegetables were tender. What should I have done?

_____

_____

3. Dear Sam,

I don't drink much milk but I love cream soups like cream of broccoli, cream of potato, and clam chowder. Can I count the milk in these soups toward the number of servings of milk I need each day?

_____

_____

4. Dear Sam,

I eat a lot of soup because it is fast and convenient and I like it. How healthful is soup? Are there ways to make it even more healthful?

_____

_____

_____

_____

CHAPTER **38** Soups

Soup Match Ups

Directions: Match each definition in the left column with the correct term from the right column. Write the letter of the term in the space provided. Do not use any term more than once. Some terms will not be used.

Definitions

____ 1. Soup that only needs to be heated and served.

____ 2. A thick soup made with vegetables, fish, or seafood.

____ 3. A flavorful liquid made by long slow cooking of meat or poultry in water.

____ 4. A soup made from cooked vegetables, meat, or poultry.

____ 5. A soup often based on white sauce.

____ 6. A clear flavorful liquid that can be made from cubes or granules.

____ 7. The liquid in soup.

Terms

A. Bouillon

B. Broth

C. Chowder

D. Convenience soup

E. Cream soup

F. Hearty soup

G. Light soup

H. Microwave soup

I. Stock

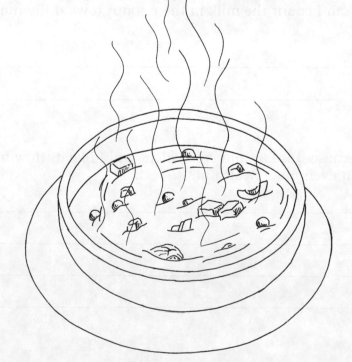

CHAPTER 39

Main Dish Mixtures

Study Guide

Directions: Answer the following questions on the lines provided.

1. Why are main dish mixtures usually economical?

   _____

   _____

   _____

2. Why does the nutritional value of main dish mixtures vary?

   _____

   _____

3. How can convenience foods be used in main dish mixtures?

   _____

   _____

   _____

4. How is stew similar to soup? How is it different?

   _____

   _____

5. What is a casserole? What ingredients are typically used in casseroles?

   _____

   _____

   _____

6. Identify three ingredients that could be added to a casserole for flavor or texture.

   _____

   _____

   _____

   _____

Continued on next page

7. What are the advantages of using a topping on a casserole? How should a casserole with a topping be baked?

_____

_____

8. What is a wok? What is it used for?

_____

_____

_____

9. What is the key to making a successful stir-fry?

_____

_____

10. Why should stir-fry ingredients be cut in small uniform pieces? Why should a stir-fry meal not be overcooked?

_____

_____

11. List three convenience products you could use in making a pizza.

_____

_____

_____

_____

12. How can you use a microwave in preparing main dish mixtures?

_____

_____

CHAPTER 39
Main Dish Mixtures

Scrambled Ingredients

Directions: Listed below in scrambled form are nine
ingredients often used in one-dish meals. Unscramble
the letters to discover the ingredient. On the lines
provided, describe how each ingredient is used in a
one-dish meal.

Scrambled Ingredients	Ingredients	Use in Main Dish Mixtures
1. vieencnoecn dosof	_____	_____
		_____
2. ohlwe risgan	_____	_____
		_____
3. ilo	_____	_____
		_____
4. lporuyt	_____	_____
		_____
5. teihw ueasc	_____	_____
		_____
6. ttoopsea	_____	_____
		_____
7. snsoagnise	_____	_____
		_____
8. gpnipsot	_____	_____
		_____
9. tysae gdohu	_____	_____

CHAPTER **39** Main Dish Mixtures

Main Dish Crossword

Directions: Fill in the crossword puzzle by placing the answers to each number below in the appropriate space.

Across

1. A food that can be used as a base for pizza. (2 words)
3. A source of protein in casseroles. (2 words)
8. A type of main dish mixture made on the range. (2 words)
9. A large pan with a rounded bottom used for stir-frying.
10. A food often served with stir-fry.
11. An ingredient mixed with water for thickening.
14. An ingredient in which stir-fry is cooked.
16. Pizza crust is usually made from this. (2 words)
17. One of the last vegetables to add when stir-frying.
19. A type of main dish mixture with a crust or base, sauce, toppings, and cheese.
22. A topping for casseroles.
25. A mixture of foods baked together.
26. Main dish mixtures can be cooked on this appliance.
29. A common ingredient in stir-frying.
31. A type of protein convenience food used in one-dish meals. (2 words)
32. One step in using ground meat or poultry in a casserole.
33. A kind of vegetable often used in stir-frying.
34. A nutrient often supplied by main dish mixtures.

Down

1. Whole grains provide this in one-dish meals.
2. A type of pan often used to make pizza. (2 words)
4. An ingredient used as a liquid in casseroles.
5. Ingredients added to flavor main dish mixtures.
6. Cooking food quickly in hot oil. (2 words)
7. An appliance used to thaw or precook ingredients before preparing main dish mixtures.
11. May be used to reduce the preparation time of main dish mixtures. (2 words)
12. A food used to complete a meal when serving a main dish mixture.
13. A topping used on pizza.
15. Protein food used to lower fat content in main dish mixtures. (2 words)
18. A kind of cheese used on pizza.
19. Provides protein in some main dish mixtures.
20. A type of ingredient in casseroles that adds nutrients and flavor while holding iingredients together.
21. Cooking method used with a skillet meal.
23. To cut ingredients into small pieces for casseroles or stir-fry.
24. A main dish mixture similar to soup, but with less liquid.
27. A spice used to flavor some main dish mixtures.
28. One of the first ingredients to cook when stir-frying.
30. What you do to cheese before it is put on pizza.

Continued on next page

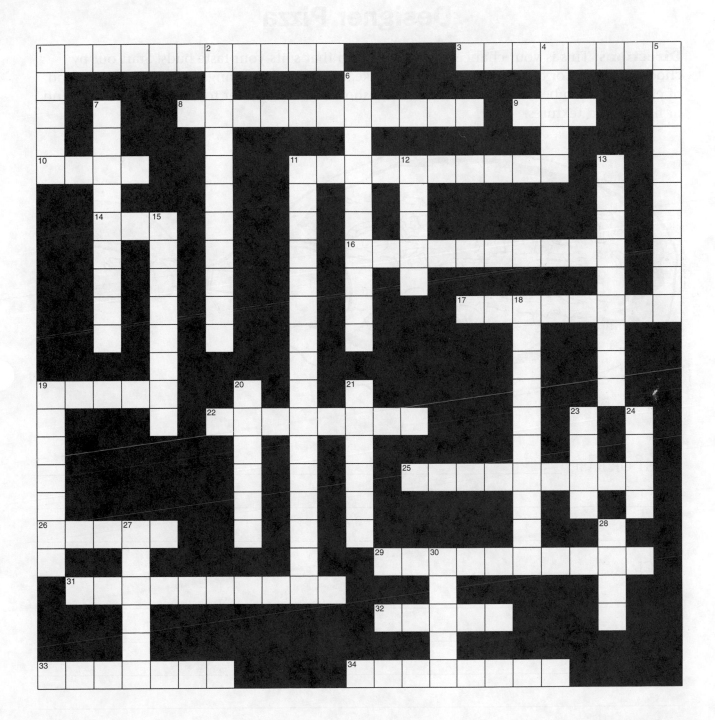

| CHAPTER **39** | Text Pages 316-323 |

Main Dish Mixtures

Designer Pizza

Directions: This is your chance to design a pizza that suits your taste buds! Start out by choosing a crust or base. Select a sauce you like, at least four toppings, and at least one kind of cheese. Remember that all the ingredients should work together to create a pleasing blend of flavors and textures.

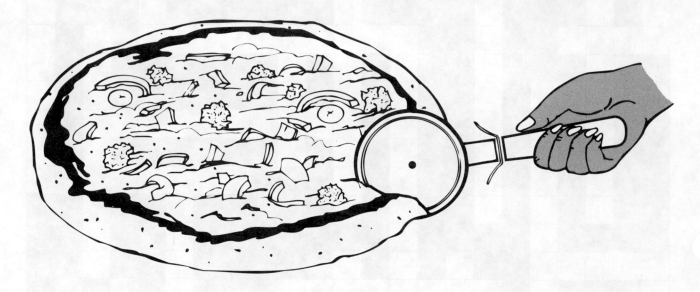

CRUST OR BASE: _____

_____

_____

SAUCE: _____

_____

_____

TOPPINGS: _____

_____

_____

_____

CHEESE: _____

_____

_____

CHAPTER 40 Snacks

Study Guide

Directions: Answer the following questions on the lines provided.

1. Why should snacks be as carefully chosen as meals?

_____

_____

2. From which of the food groups on the Food Guide Pyramid should snacks come?

_____

_____

3. Why should candy bars and chips be enjoyed as an occasional treat rather than a daily choice?

_____

_____

_____

4. Why is constant snacking not a good idea?

_____

_____

_____

5. Why should you brush your teeth after snacking whenever possible?

_____

_____

6. What kind of snacks should someone who has low energy needs choose?

_____

_____

7. How can you be sure the snacks you eat fit into your total eating plan?

_____

_____

_____

Continued on next page

8. Why should you read the nutrition labels when selecting snacks?

_____

_____

9. How can spreads be used as snacks?

_____

_____

10. Why is popcorn considered an ideal snack? How can you flavor air-popped popcorn without adding fat or salt?

_____

_____

_____

11. Why do fruits and vegetables make good snacks?

_____

_____

12. Name at least four other healthful snack ideas. How could you use the microwave oven to help you prepare snacks?

_____

_____

_____

_____

_____

_____

CHAPTER 40 Snacks

Vending Machine Choices

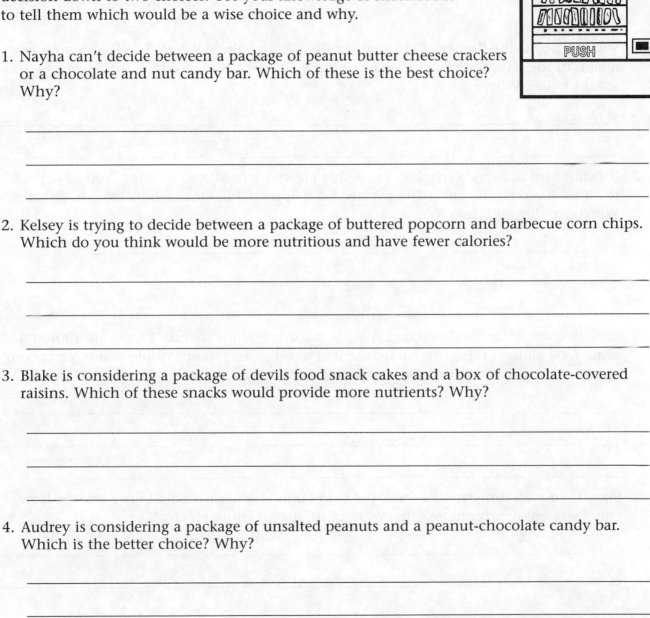

Directions: You and some friends are at a vending machine to buy after school snacks. In each case, your friends have narrowed the decision down to two choices. Use your knowledge of snack foods to tell them which would be a wise choice and why.

1. Nayha can't decide between a package of peanut butter cheese crackers or a chocolate and nut candy bar. Which of these is the best choice? Why?

_____

_____

_____

2. Kelsey is trying to decide between a package of buttered popcorn and barbecue corn chips. Which do you think would be more nutritious and have fewer calories?

_____

_____

3. Blake is considering a package of devils food snack cakes and a box of chocolate-covered raisins. Which of these snacks would provide more nutrients? Why?

_____

_____

_____

4. Audrey is considering a package of unsalted peanuts and a peanut-chocolate candy bar. Which is the better choice? Why?

_____

_____

_____

Name _____ Date _____ Class Period _____

Great Snacks

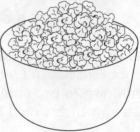

Directions: Read each situation described below. Answer the questions on the lines provided.

1. You will be having dinner in less than an hour, but you're starving. You find some watermelon in the refrigerator and brownies on the kitchen counter. Which would be a better snack choice? Why?

_____

_____

2. It's your turn to bring a snack to eat during an after-school club meeting. You have potato chips, pretzels, and chocolate-covered pretzels on hand. One club member is diabetic. Which would you bring? Why?

_____

_____

3. You are going to an outdoor concert at the park with some friends. People are allowed to bring food along, or they may purchase it at a concession stand. Would you buy popcorn or bring your own? Several of you are watching your fat intake closely.

_____

_____

4. Pizza is your all-time favorite food, but your family has it only about once a week. How could you enjoy pizza more often without baking an entire pizza?

_____

_____

5. If you were trying to choose healthful snacks to eat, what characteristics would you look for?

_____

_____

Name _____ Date _____ Class Period _____

CHAPTER 41

Beverages

Study Guide

Directions: Answer the following questions on the lines provided.

1. What is the best beverage for quenching thirst?

_____

2. Why is it important to include milk as a regular beverage in your diet?

_____

_____

3. Are milk shakes as nutritious as plain milk? Why or why not?

_____

_____

4. Why should coffee, tea, and soft drinks be used only as an occasional treat, not as part of the regular diet?

_____

_____

5. Why is it best to avoid drinks that contain caffeine?

_____

_____

6. A bottle of juice is labeled "10 percent juice." If there are 10 cups in the bottle, how many cups are pure juice?

_____

7. What does it mean when the directions of a frozen juice concentrate says to reconstitute the juice?

_____

_____

Continued on next page

8. Which of the following are forms of sugars: fructose, corn syrup, honey, dextrose, and sucrose?

_____

_____

9. The label of a bottle of orange drink lists the ingredients as: Water, Fructose, Orange Juice, Coloring. Does this contain more water, sugar, or juice? Explain your answer.

_____

_____

_____

10. How should you choose which juices to combine to make a fruit punch?

_____

_____

11. How can you make blender shakes that will be a nutritious snack?

_____

_____

_____

12. Why should you pay careful attention to beverages that are heated in the microwave?

_____

_____

CHAPTER 41

Beverages

Where's the Juice?

Directions: Where should a shopper look for juices in the supermarket? Match each beverage in the left column with the correct location in the supermarket from the right column. Write the letter of the location in the space provided. Each location will be used at least once.

Beverages

____ 1. Powdered orange drink mix

____ 2. Canned tomato juice

____ 3. Bottle of cranberry-apple juice

____ 4. Frozen pineapple juice concentrate

____ 5. Fresh grapefruit juice

____ 6. Individual boxes of grape juice

____ 7. Canned vegetable juice

____ 8. Fresh orange juice

____ 9. Canned grapefruit juice

____ 10. Individual boxes of apple juice

____ 11. Frozen grape juice concentrate

____ 12. Canned apricot nectar

Supermarket Locations

A. Frozen section

B. Grocery shelves

C. Refrigerated section

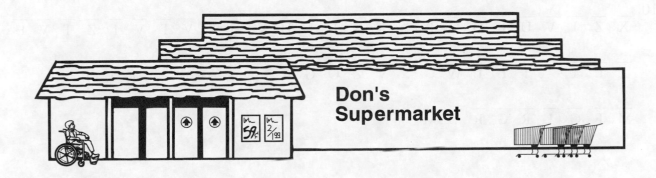

Don's Supermarket

CHAPTER 41

Beverages

Coded Messages

Directions: The following sentences contain coded terms from the chapter. Use the example and the sentences to break the code. Then decode the mystery message in number 10.

Example: $\underline{B}\ \underline{E}\ \underline{V}\ \underline{E}\ \underline{R}\ \underline{A}\ \underline{G}\ \underline{E}\ \underline{S}$
$\ \underline{Y}\ \underline{V}\ \underline{E}\ \underline{V}\ \underline{I}\ \underline{Z}\ \underline{T}\ \underline{V}\ \underline{H}$

1. Sometimes a mixture of fruit juices is called a $\underline{\ }\ \underline{\ }\ \underline{\ }\ \underline{\ }\ \underline{\ }\quad \underline{\ }\ \underline{\ }\ \underline{\ }\ \underline{\ }\ \underline{\ }.$
   $ U\ I\ F\ R\ G\quad K\ F\ M\ X\ S$

2. A beverage high in potassium and vitamin C is $\underline{\ }\ \underline{\ }\ \underline{\ }\ \underline{\ }\ \underline{\ }\quad \underline{\ }\ \underline{\ }\ \underline{\ }\ \underline{\ }.$
   $ L\ I\ Z\ M\ T\ V\quad Q\ F\ R\ X\ V$

3. The only way to know exactly what is in a beverage container is to

   $\underline{\ }\ \underline{\ }\ \underline{\ }\ \underline{\ }\quad \underline{\ }\ \underline{\ }\ \underline{\ }\quad \underline{\ }\ \underline{\ }\ \underline{\ }\ \underline{\ }.$
   $I\ V\ Z\ W\quad G\ S\ V\quad O\ Z\ Y\ V\ O$

4. Coffee and tea contain $\underline{\ }\ \underline{\ }\ \underline{\ }\ \underline{\ }\ \underline{\ }\ \underline{\ }\ \underline{\ }\ \underline{\ }$ that can stimulate the nervous
   $ X\ Z\ U\ U\ V\ R\ M\ V$ system.

5. Drinking $\underline{\ }\ \underline{\ }\ \underline{\ }\ \underline{\ }\ \underline{\ }$ is the best way to quench a thirst.
   $ D\ Z\ G\ V\ I$

6. A product that contains some juice with water and sweeteners is called a

   $\underline{\ }\ \underline{\ }\ \underline{\ }\ \underline{\ }\quad \underline{\ }\ \underline{\ }\ \underline{\ }\ \underline{\ }.$
   $U\ I\ F\ R\ G\quad W\ I\ R\ M\ P$

7. Drinking $\underline{\ }\ \underline{\ }\ \underline{\ }\ \underline{\ }$ provides vitamins A and D.
   $ N\ R\ O\ P$

8. Regular soft drinks contain lots of $\underline{\ }\ \underline{\ }\ \underline{\ }\ \underline{\ }\ \underline{\ }.$
   $ H\ F\ T\ Z\ I$

9. Until you are ready to use them, keep fruit juice concentrates $\underline{\ }\ \underline{\ }\ \underline{\ }\ \underline{\ }\ \underline{\ }\ \underline{\ }.$
   $ U\ I\ L\ A\ V\ M$

10. $\underline{\ }\ \underline{\ }\ \underline{\ }\ \underline{\ }\ \underline{\ }\ \underline{\ }\ \underline{\ }\ \underline{\ }\ \underline{\ }\quad \underline{\ }\ \underline{\ }\ \underline{\ }\ \underline{\ }\ \underline{\ }\quad \underline{\ }\ \underline{\ }\ \underline{\ }\ \underline{\ }\ \underline{\ }\ \underline{\ }\ \underline{\ }\ \underline{\ }\ \underline{\ }$
    $X\ Z\ I\ V\ U\ F\ O\ O\ B\quad X\ S\ L\ L\ H\ V\quad Y\ V\ E\ V\ I\ Z\ T\ V\ H$

    $\underline{\ }\ \underline{\ }\ \underline{\ }\quad \underline{\ }\ \underline{\ }\ \underline{\ }\ \underline{\ }\quad \underline{\ }\ \underline{\ }\ \underline{\ }\ \underline{\ }\ \underline{\ }\quad \underline{\ }\ \underline{\ }\ \underline{\ }\quad \underline{\ }\ \underline{\ }\ \underline{\ }\ \underline{\ }$
    $U\ L\ I\quad T\ L\ L\ W\quad S\ V\ Z\ O\ G\ S\quad Z\ M\ W\quad T\ L\ L\ W$

    $\underline{\ }\ \underline{\ }\ \underline{\ }\ \underline{\ }\ \underline{\ }\ \underline{\ }\ \underline{\ }\ \underline{\ }.$
    $M\ F\ G\ I\ R\ G\ R\ L\ M$

CHAPTER 42 Principles of Baking

Study Guide

Directions: Answer the following questions on the lines provided.

1. Why is a recipe like a chemical formula?

_____

_____

_____

_____

2. Why is flour an essential ingredient in baked goods?

_____

_____

3. How do leavening agents work?

_____

_____

4. Why are baked goods so different from each other when they are made from basically the same ingredients?

_____

_____

5. What is the mixture of ingredients called when making pancakes?

_____

6. What are the four types of leavening agents? What is the source of each?

_____

_____

_____

_____

Continued on next page

7. Why is it important to follow the recipe when making a baked product?

_____

_____

_____

8. What will happen if you substitute melted butter for solid shortening in a cookie recipe?

_____

_____

9. Why do some recipes call for greased and floured pans?

_____

_____

_____

10. What adjustments, if any, should be made to the oven temperature given in the recipe if you are using a shiny metal pan? A glass pan?

_____

_____

11. Why should baking pans have the bottoms and sides wiped before being put in the oven?

_____

_____

12. What equipment or tool should be used to cool baked goods?

_____

CHAPTER 42   Principles of Baking

STEPS to Baking Success

Directions: Five important steps in successful baking are listed on the stair steps below. On the lines provided, explain why each step is important in baking success.

5. Use the correct oven temperature. Why?

_____

_____

_____

4. Use the correct type and size of pan. Why?

_____

_____

_____

3. Follow the directions in the recipe. Why?

_____

_____

_____

2. Measure accurately. Why?

_____

_____

_____

1. Use the exact ingredients called for in the recipe. Why?

_____

_____

_____

Principles of Baking

Analyzing Recipe Ingredients

Directions: In the chart on the next page, the seven categories of ingredients commonly used in baking are listed on the left. Write the purpose of each ingredient in the spaces provided. Then read the ingredient list for Pineapple-Pecan Bread. Write the name or names of the ingredient that is an example of the ingredient category in the recipe.

 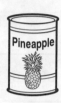 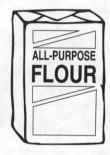 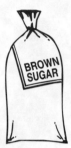 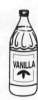

Pineapple-Pecan Bread

1/2 cup brown sugar

1/4 cup butter or margarine

1 egg

2 cups all-purpose flour

1 tsp. baking soda

1/3 cup frozen orange
  juice concentrate, thawed

3 Tbsp. water

1 8.5-oz. can crushed pineapple,
  undrained

1 tsp. vanilla

1/2 cup chopped pecans

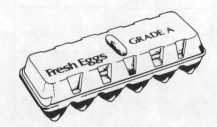

Continued on next page

Ingredient Category	Purpose of Ingredient in Recipe	Example(s) of Ingredient Category in Pineapple-Pecan Bread
Flour	1.	8.
Leavening Agent	2.	9.
Liquid	3.	10.
Fat/Oil	4.	11.
Sweetener	5.	12.
Eggs	6.	13.
Flavoring	7.	14.

CHAPTER 42

Text Pages 340-347

Principles of Baking

Preparing to Bake

Directions: Assume you are preparing to bake a layer cake. The recipe tells you to prepare the baking pans. Listed below are the steps to follow when preparing a cake pan for baking. Place a 1 in the blank to the left of the first step in preparing a cake pan. Place a 2 in the blank to the left of the second step. Continue until all steps are numbered in order.

____ 1. Hold the pan in both hands, gently turning it to spread the flour evenly over the bottom and sides of the pan.

____ 2. Using waxed paper or a paper towel, spread shortening in a thin, even layer over the bottom and sides of the pan.

____ 3. Turn the pan upside down.

____ 4. Sprinkle about 1 tablespoon of flour over the pan.

____ 5. Hold the pan over a large piece of waxed paper.

____ 6. Tap the pan gently to remove excess flour.

____ 7. Tap the pan gently to spread the flour.

Directions: The cake recipe you are using says that the cake batter can be baked in two round 8 x 1½ inch cake pans or in one rectangular 9 x 13 x 2 inch cake pan. On the oven rack drawings below, draw the placement of the cake pans for baking using both the round pans and the rectangular pan.

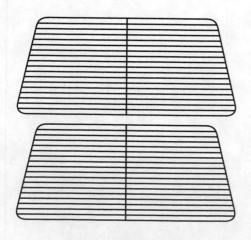

Round Cake Pans

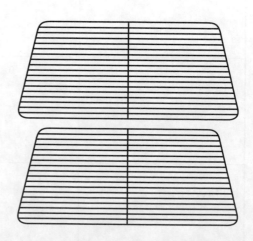

Rectangular Cake Pan

CHAPTER **43**
Baking Breads

Study Guide

Directions: Answer the following questions on the lines provided.

1. What makes a bread a quick bread?

_____

_____

2. What is the difference between regular flour and self-rising flour?

_____

_____

3. What happens if you make a product with baking powder after its "use by" date?

_____

_____

4. Which fat or oil should be used if you wanted to reduce the amount of saturated fat in a baked product?

_____

5. Why is yeast dough set aside before baking?

_____

_____

6. Describe the muffin method of making pancakes.

_____

_____

_____

7. How should the crust of a quick bread look when it is finished baking?

_____

_____

Continued on next page

8. Why is a different method used to prepare biscuits than to prepare muffins?

_____

_____

9. How long should biscuit dough be kneaded? What happens if it is kneaded too long?

_____

_____

10. What does dry yeast need to produce gas to make dough rise?

_____

_____

11. What produces the tiny holes in baked bread or rolls?

_____

_____

12. What type of pan gives the best results when making quick breads in the microwave?

_____

_____

Name _____ Date _____ Class Period _____

Mixing Methods

Directions: The steps in the muffin and biscuit methods of making quick breads are mixed up in the muffins and biscuits below. Identify which step belongs to which mixing method and write the steps in the proper order on the blanks below.

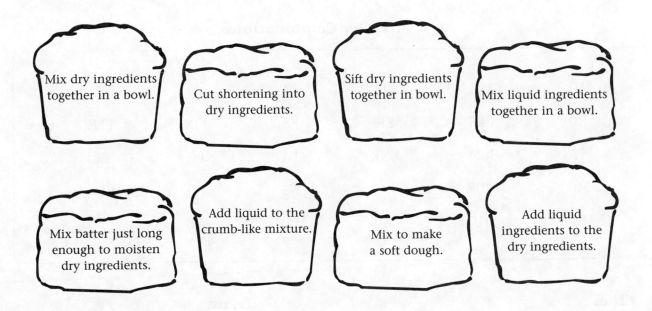

Mix dry ingredients together in a bowl.

Cut shortening into dry ingredients.

Sift dry ingredients together in bowl.

Mix liquid ingredients together in a bowl.

Mix batter just long enough to moisten dry ingredients.

Add liquid to the crumb-like mixture.

Mix to make a soft dough.

Add liquid ingredients to the dry ingredients.

Muffin Method	Biscuit Method
1.	1.
2.	2.
3.	3.
4.	4.

| CHAPTER **43** | | Text Pages 348-357 |

Baking Breads

Quick Bread Combinations

Directions: Put together letter combinations from the list below to form terms from Chapter 43. Use the clues and the letter combinations to help you discover the terms. Cross off the letter combinations in the list as you use them.

List of Letter Combinations

AD	AVE	BIS	CA	CO	CU
ED	ELS	ER	ES	FIN	FLE
IT	IUM	KNE	LA	LC	LE
MO	MUF	NN	NS	PO	RED
SS	TU	VE	WAF	WD	

Clues   **Terms**

1. To work or press dough with the hands. _____

2. A type of quick bread. _____

3. A method for mixing quick breads. _____

4. What baking powder does for quick breads. _____

5. Mineral in bread provided by milk. _____

6. A result of overmixing. _____

7. The kind of container in which flour is stored. _____

8. A method for mixing quick breads. _____

9. An ingredient in brown sugar. _____

10. Sugar that has a fine texture. _____

CHAPTER 44

Cookies, Cakes, and Pies

Study Guide

Directions: Answer the following questions on the lines provided.

1. Identify two types of convenience cookies that will save preparation time.

   _____

2. How should cream pies be stored? Why?

   _____

   _____

3. What is the difference between drop and molded cookies?

   _____

   _____

4. What are the similarities and differences between rolled and refrigerator cookies?

   _____

   _____

   _____

5. How do you know when cookies are done baking?

   _____

   _____

6. What leavening is used in foam cakes?

   _____

   _____

7. Why are some cakes baked in a tube pan?

   _____

   _____

Continued on next page

8. What qualities are found in a properly baked cake?

_____

_____

9. What equipment or tools would you need to remove a cake from its pan?

_____

_____

10. What ingredients are used to make pastry for pie? What is the main quality of a good pastry?

_____

_____

11. What is a chiffon pie?

_____

_____

_____

12. How does *convection* baking differ from conventional baking?

_____

_____

_____

CHAPTER 44

Cookies, Cakes, and Pies

Problem Solvers

Directions: Read the situations below. Answer the questions on the lines provided.

1. Sean bought a ready-made graham cracker pie crust. How will he know how to store it?

_____

_____

_____

2. Carlotta is on a low-fat diet. She allows herself one dessert treat a week. What are two sweets that are relatively low in fat?

_____

_____

_____

3. Paul wants to make a pie to serve his friends, but he only has an hour before they arrive. All the recipes he checks take too long. What could he do?

_____

_____

_____

4. Rakeisha is making rolled gingerbread cookies, but the dough keeps sticking to her rolling pin and the cookie cutter. What should she do?

_____

_____

_____

Continued on next page

Chapter 44: Cookies, Cakes, and Pies (*Continued*)

5. Narmar made oatmeal cookies. Some were thick and chewy while others were thin, crisp, and very brown. What could Narmar have done to prevent this?

_____

_____

_____

_____

6. Abby was making a batch of molded lemon cookies. She was refilling the baking sheet as soon as she removed the baked cookies. Many of her cookies were very spread out and thin. What could have prevented this?

_____

_____

_____

_____

7. Ryne made an angel food cake. When he went to take it out of the pan, it had fallen and was very thin. How could he have prevented this from happening?

_____

_____

_____

_____

8. Minh baked a pan of brownies in a square pan in the microwave. The corners were burned and hard and couldn't be eaten. Why did this happen? How could Minh have prevented it?

_____

_____

_____

_____

CHAPTER 44

Cookies, Cakes, and Pies

Sweet Treat Match Ups

Directions: Match each description or example in the left column with the correct type of cookie from the right column. Write the letter of the type of cookie in the space provided. Each type of cookie will be used at least once.

Description or Example	Type of Cookie
____ 1. Sliced from a long roll of chilled dough.	A. Bar
____ 2. Peanut butter cookies.	B. Drop
____ 3. Shaped from a stiff dough with a cookie press.	C. Molded
____ 4. Shaped by dropping batter on a baking sheet.	D. Pressed
____ 5. Made from stiff dough with cookie cutters.	E. Refrigerator
____ 6. Brownies.	F. Rolled
____ 7. Spritz cookies.	
____ 8. Baked in a square or rectangular pan and cut into shapes.	
____ 9. Shaped by hand from a stiff dough.	
____ 10. Sugar cookies.	

Continued on next page

Chapter 44: Sweet Treat Match Ups (*Continued*)

Directions: Match each description or example in the left column with the correct type of pie from the right column. Write the letter of the type of pie in the space provided. Each type of pie will be used at least once.

Description or Example

____ 11. Coconut cream

____ 12. Lemon meringue

____ 13. Has only a top crust with a fruit fillin.

____ 14. Has a filling between a top and bottom crust

____ 15. Blueberry pie

____ 16. Has a bottom crust with a filling

Type of Pie

A. Two-crust pie

B. One-crust pie

C. Deep-dish pie

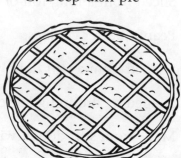

Directions: Match each description or example in the left column with the correct types of cake from the right column. Write the letter of the type of pie in the space provided.

Description or Example

____ 17. A cake that does not contain fat or oil.

____ 18. A cake that contains fat, such as shortening or margarine.

____ 19. A cake that contains baking powder or soda for leavening.

____ 20. A cake that is baked in a tube pan.

Type of Cake

A. Shortened cakes

B. Unshortened cakes

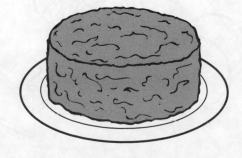
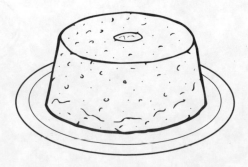